THE MEN
BEHIND
HITLER

A GERMAN WARNING
TO THE WORLD

BERNHARD SCHREIBER

THE MEN BEHIND HITLER

A GERMAN WARNING TO THE WORLD

BERNHARD SCHREIBER

Suzeteo Enterprises

The Men Behind Hitler:
A German warning to the world
by Bernhard Schreiber
Translated by H.R. Martindale

ISBN 978-1-947844-48-3
Published by Suzeteo Enterprises.
Copyright 2018, All Rights Reserved.

A note from the Editor: As best as can be ascertained, H.R. Martindale translated Schreiber's writing as well as the German documents included in the appendix. A statement in Schreiber's book, by the author, indicates that the entire book is free for reproduction and redistribution. However, a translation was not provided for Dr. Hoff's Foreword (pages 124-125), so Suzeteo Enterprises has obtained one by Dr. Kirk Allison. This translation is copyrighted, and cannot be reproduced without permission.]

For more information about eugenics and the subject matter of this book, visit www.eugenics.us.

TABLE OF CONTENTS

Items in the Appendix:
Sterilization in the United States to 1956
The Eugenics Education Society Board 1915-1916
The "Scientific" Works on which Professor Lenz bases his work.
Archiv für Rassenhygiene. (English and German)
On the Occasion of Hitler's Birthday (English and German)
The War Forced Upon Us and Racial Hygiene (English and German)
The Perfection of Great Germany (English and German)
Duties and Aims of the German Society for Racial Hygiene (English and German)
The Führer thanks Rüdin. (English and German)
The Relation of National Socialism to Racial Hygiene (English and German)
Photos [T4 transport list; Dr. Karl Brandt; concentration camps; etc.]
The National Council for Mental Hygiene [Various lists]
Vorwort — Hoff's Preface to the book "Euthanasia and the Destruction of 'Life Unworthy' Life" by Helmut Ehrhardt. (English and German)
Proponents of Legalizing Euthanasia
Proponents of Abortion on Demand and Birth Control
The Relation of National Socialism to Racial Hygiene by Dr. Lenz (English and German)
A Final Tribute to Ploetz (English and German)
World Federation for Mental Health Member List
Included in Schreiber's original book but available only online at www.eugenics.us:
Strategic Planning for Mental Health. By Colonel J. R. Rees, M.D.
The Concept and Prevalence of Mental Retardation by T.L Pilkington

Bernhard Schreiber was born in 1942 in Stuttgart after his father died in action as an officer of the Luftwaffe. After his education in Germany he studied journalism in America and travelled extensively as a freelance journalist.

DEDICATION

This book is humbly dedicated to the memory of countless ordinary people — those men, women, children and babies of many races and beliefs, whose lives were taken because they were considered less than perfect and, therefore, unworthy to live.

I hope that this small book will serve in its own way to keep their memory alive and that it will help to remind us all of the price we have to pay when extremists have the power to decide upon our right to live.

Bernhard Schreiber

Foreword

by Dr. Anthony Horvath

1.

My investigation into these matters began after my wife and I were counseled to abort our daughter, diagnosed in the womb a few minutes earlier with spina bifida. A few weeks later, I felt a deep need to understand how a doctor could put a question like that to a couple thrown into such turmoil and confusion. A book like Bernhard Schreiber's would have answered almost all of my questions in a single shot if I had been aware of it. That said, *The Men Behind Hitler* is almost unbelievable if you don't have some other reason to suspect what is going on.

Long story short, I did not have Schreiber's book. I had to piece it together for myself. In the ten years of research that followed, I acquired hundreds of primary sources and probably as many secondary sources, as well as my doctorate, which was heavily orientated towards a study of eugenics and evolutionary ethics.

With that experience, I can usually tell who has taken the time to study the matter. The general outline of their telling of the story is roughly the same: it begins with Malthus, passes through Darwin, then Galton, at which point it branches out into the international community where the story fractures into pieces and takes on different characteristics depending on what country accepted the starting premises.

Schreiber's emphasis, as one might expect, is on how the premises manifested in his native country of Germany, and then, as he will tell you himself, how he witnessed it unfold in the United Kingdom. My own understanding of the story was viewed through the prism of the United States. However, anyone who goes on this particular quest comes to realize very early on that the whole story requires looking beyond one's own borders. Most of the world was on roughly the same track until Germany ruined it by exposing in the short span of a decade or so just how wretched things could go for people who really tried to live according to the starting principles.

After that, the various storylines converge again: it is no longer fashionable to openly say the things that were said by nearly all of the mainstream scientists prior to 1940, and, to be fair, many of the proponents of these 'eugenic' philosophies did a bit of soul-searching, wondering to themselves how things could have gone so badly.

People who continue to follow the story observe that these various proponents and their respective organizations change their tactics. They go 'crypto.' They change their names and sometimes re-label their mission so it is more palatable to their communities, and perhaps their own consciences. Moreover, they more or less abandon any of their talk about 'compulsory' measures, and begin focusing on 'voluntary' proposals.

Enter the psychiatrists and propagandists, who will do their part to get people to decide to behave 'eugenically' and think it is their own idea, and of course, for the common good. In the immortal words of Frederick Osborn in 1956:

> People will accept the idea of a specific hereditary defect. They will go to a heredity clinic and ask what is the risk of our having a defective child. They balance that risk against the chance of their having a sound child, and they usually come up with a pretty sound decision. But they won't accept the idea that they are in general second rate. We must rely on other motivation.

> Given the right circumstances, people will have children in proportion to their ability to care for them. If they feel financially secure, if they enjoy accepting responsibility, if they have warm affectional responses, if they are physically strong and competent, they are likely to

have large families, **provided they have a reasonable psychological conditioning** to this end. If they are unable to feed the children they have, if they are afraid of responsibility, if their affectional responses are weak, people don't want many children. If they have effective means of family planning, they won't have many. Our studies have shown this to be true all over the world. On such a base it is surely possible to build a system of **voluntary unconscious selection.**[1] [Emphasis added]

In other words, with the right 'psychological conditioning' you can get people to apply Darwinian selection in their own families and think it is their own idea, without knowing that the ideas actually are the regurgitated, re-made, re-packaged, and re-distributed guiding principles that drove the eugenics movement on in the early 20th century.

This, more or less, became the policy of these proponents, if only because it was the only remaining option they saw that might bring them success.

As one might expect, the story has continued to progress since the mid-1970s when Schreiber wrote this book. On top of that, as Schreiber readily admits, there were many other avenues to explore beyond what he presented. However, he brought something to the table that many researchers lack, and that is the ability to speak German. His ability to access the writings of those in Germany allowed him to document more of the ideological history of Hitler and the Nazis. He was then able to connect those ideas and individuals with those elsewhere--such as in the United Kingdom-- who had many of the same ideas.

The problem, if the reader doesn't see it instinctively, is that the Nazis are roundly condemned, whereas those who had many of the same ideas and were actively trying to implement them in their own way in their own nations, have been not only been able to do so with relative impunity, hardly anyone even knows what they were about. To the degree that anyone does know their names, their reputations are fully intact.

---

[1] Frederick Osborn in his Galton Lecture of 1956, titled "Galton and Mid-Century Eugenics" as found in the April 1956 edition of *The Eugenics Review*.

But Schreiber draws the same conclusion that many other researchers draw: it is reasonable to believe that the same bitter roots will yield the same bitter fruits.

That doesn't mean that he, or I, know what form that this will take. Now some fifty years after Schreiber wrote, we have a broader perspective in analyzing that question. Still, any analysis would require being aware of the basic outline that he set out to present to readers. The reader can be assured that, in the main, Schreiber's research 'checks out.' If, after reading this book, you feel a sense of foreboding, you are on the right track. But that is nothing compared to the foreboding you will feel if you pick up the threads yourself and begin researching the matter for yourself. The prospects for the future, grounded as they are on the successful implementation of the 'psychological conditioning' that Osborn keenly desired, do not bode well.

2.

I have intentionally tried to refrain from adding too much to Schreiber's account because, as I said, the truth of the matter is so nefarious that it is frankly unbelievable unless you see the evidence for yourself. If I had not personally been in the room when a doctor instantly proposed abortion as an appropriate response to the diagnosis of a birth defect, I don't think I could have believed it, myself. Nor could I have believed the implications of the research I turned up later.

As one reads Schreiber's book (or even any of my own writings), it will be tempting to console oneself by suggesting that while these various remarks that have been documented do indeed have a sinister taint to them, they are probably just outliers or taken out of context, etc. The truth is that for every source given, hundreds more could be provided. The constraints of publication and communication in general require narrowing the case down to a select number of sources. The reader should not make the mistake of thinking that Schreiber has fixed upon an exception. The scary truth is that the examples he give are representative of the general current of scholarship and thinking both within Germany and out, in the 1930s and later when he was writing in the 1970s.

One can almost see that Schreiber is aware that people will try to dismiss his book for the simple reason that it focuses on just thirty people or so. He packed the book's appendix with so many reproductions of primary source material that it nearly doubled the length of his overall book. I suspect he did this so that the reader could see just how many names there are associated with the eugenics philosophies Schreiber referenced.

Schreiber wants the reader to notice how many of these names appear on multiple lists: the same individuals who advocate for 'voluntary' euthanasia are also members of a eugenics society, as well as proponents of abortion on demand, and of course 'mental hygiene.' In other words, these people themselves understood that their mindset required them to be involved in dozens of different projects.

The reader may not understand the connections between these projects until they've done a bit more research, but these individuals themselves surely did.

To illustrate, once again, consider this quote by the above mentioned Frederick Osborn:

> Birth control and abortion are turning out to be great eugenic advances of our time. If they had been advanced for eugenic reasons it would have retarded or stopped their acceptance.[2]

In my experience, very few people, especially advocates for abortion on demand, see birth control or abortion as having anything whatsoever to do with eugenics. This is a good example of what Colonel Rees[3] had in mind when he said,

> If we are to infiltrate the professional and social activities of other people I think we must imitate the Totalitarian and organise some kind of fifth column activity! If better ideas on mental health are to progress and spread we, as the salesmen, must lose our identity. By that I mean that we cannot help so effectively if speaking for a National Council or any other body as we can when we make a more subtle approach adapted to the particular

---

[2] http://eugenics.us/frederick-osborn-birth-control-and-abortion-are-turning-out-to-be-great-eugenic-advances/256.htm

[3] See Chapter 8.

circumstances of the moment. **It really wouldn't matter if no one ever heard of this Council again provided that the work was done.** Let us all, therefore, very secretly be "fifth columnists." [Emphasis added]

Do you see it? It does not matter to them that other people do not see what they are doing as 'eugenics' *so long as they are doing it.* So, too, Osborn is perfectly happy to distance the eugenics movement from abortion on demand since he knows that nonetheless, abortion on demand is one of the "great eugenics advances of our time."

Now keep your eyes peeled for all of the different agendas they wanted to advance, knowing full well they could not be honest about their controlling ideology.[4] The astute reader will recognize that it is no longer enough to simply take a public policy on its face when *these* people are involved in it. Maximum discernment is required.

But to have that discernment, you will have to knuckle down and do a ton of research. Don't wait for tomorrow. Start today.

3.

I discovered *The Men Behind Hitler* in the spring of 2018 during the natural course of my own continued research. Schreiber was briefly mentioned in N. D. A. Kemp's *Merciful Release: The history of the British euthanasia movement.*[5]

The mention wasn't particularly flattering, although it did acknowledge that Schreiber contributed valid insight into the German side of the question. I decided that I needed to see Schreiber's book for myself. I quickly discovered that the book was out of print.

Fortunately, the text had been reproduced on the internet in numerous places. I was especially impressed by how Liz Toolan presented it on her website. The text posted by Toolan suggested

---

[4] See also the "Jaffe Memo." www.jaffememo.com

[5] Having now read Schreiber's book, Kemp's criticism is confusing. He says that Schreiber asked "whether Nazi medical crimes could have occurred elsewhere." Does Kemp think that Schreiber believes that Jews were as likely to be rounded up in the UK as in Germany? It almost seems that Kemp takes this sentiment from the Trevor-Roper back cover blurb (below) rather than Schreiber himself. Kemp is fully aware of the ideological roots of eugenics and the many interconnections it entails, so the confusion does not seem to be one of incredulity.

that there was even more material in Schreiber's book which was not on the website, which I wanted to see as well. I emailed inquiries, but never received a reply. I decided I needed to acquire my own copy, which I did.

Therein, I discovered something else. Namely, that the author specifically encourages people to more widely distribute his book.

Being a publisher that takes a particular interest in the subject matter, and the author explicitly gave permission to reproduce the book, I decided that I needed to close the gap between 'out of print' and 'more widely distributed.' The work you hold in your hands now is my attempt to close that gap.

In general, this edition is a close reproduction of the original (in English) by Schreiber.[6] Very few updates were made. Certain Anglicisms were removed, while others were retained. Typos were corrected when discovered. There probably are even more that have been missed, and are preserved in this text. The cover, as one would expect, needed a complete overhaul, which was provided.

It seemed better to simply scan in the many items that Schreiber included in his appendix rather than attempt to re-create them. The image quality in the original wasn't that great to begin with, so the reader is duly warned that they will have to look at some of them closely in order to understand them.

Effort was made to ensure that the book and its contents were freely available to reproduce legally. The bulk of the book was easy enough--Schreiber explicitly encourages people to reproduce it. The items in the appendix are offered without many clues about their original source. A good faith effort was made to ensure that all the items that Schreiber included in his original book can be legitimately included in this edition; as the vast majority of them can be justified on a 'fair use' basis alone, there isn't much concern about that.

There are two important exceptions, however.

Schreiber includes the full text for the following two papers:

Strategic Planning for Mental Health. By Colonel J. R. Rees, M.D. and *The Concept and Prevalence of Mental Retardation* by T.L Pilkington.

I was not able to ascertain for sure that we were permitted to reproduce them in their entirety, so we did not follow Schreiber in including them in this edition.

---

[6] "Supplied" by H & P Tadeusz, London.

However, both texts can be freely found online in their entirety. If the reader wishes to read them, they can be found quickly enough by visiting www.eugenics.us[7] where both can be found.

4.

The original back cover includes a blurb by Hugh Trevor-Roper of *The Sunday Times*. It illustrates nicely what I mean about people finding this all to be unbelievable if one hasn't already done a fair bit of research:

> "The Final Solution," the systematic extermination of the Jews of Europe, is one of the most tormenting aspect of Hitler's Germany. We cannot escape from it. All easy generlisations about Nazism break upon it. So do all attempts to see the Second World War as a continuation of the first. Anti-Semitism was not a mere top-dressing of Nazism" it was central to it. The Final Solution was not an extra in Hitler's war: he was prepared to be defeated by the Allies rather than fail to destroy the Jews.
>
> How was such a programme conceivable? By what process were Germans psychologically conditioned to acquiesce in this cold-blooded, scientific barbarism? It is said that anti-Semitism has long been endemic among Germans: that in Hitler it reached paranoid proportions" and that out of their docility his fanaticism was able to forge the necessary instrument, the SS. This answer is reassuring. It implies that Germans are in some way unique: that such things cannot happen elsewhere. Such reassurance seemed to me unsoundly based.
>
> I was recently sent a little book by a German author which offers a different explanation. The explanation does not convince me, but the facts are interesting and the suggestions deserve to be pondered. The author is Bernhard Schreiber and the book is called *The Men Behind Hitler*.

---

[7] Incidentally, eugenics.us is a site that I maintain as a repository for my own research.

It is certainly true that there was something about the German nation as it emerged out of the ashes of the first World War that made it susceptible for what was to come in a manner that wasn't true about other nations. But does that mean that "such things cannot happen elsewhere"?

Like Trevor-Roper, I think there is little reason to accept such a proposition. Schreiber, certainly, would have rejected it. It is interesting, though, that so many people, after they've looked into it, chart out a similar sequence and narrative, with so many others, like Trevor-Roper, looking at the same "facts and suggestions" just can't bring themselves to be convinced.

Can such things happen elsewhere?

If they do happen again, you can be sure that one of the underlying factors uncovered will be that victims and perpetrators alike believed "it could not happen here."[8]

However, neither Schreiber nor any other researcher believes that the 'thing that could happen' is likely to be a Nazi-style elimination of the Jews, occurring in the United States or Europe. (But you would be a fool to think 'civilized' humanity is incapable of it! 'Not likely' does not mean 'impossible.')

What is deemed more likely to happen?

I've already sketched out some ideas (such as 'voluntary unconscious selection') but to be fair to the historical record, even those living through the events that manifested in the Holocaust and T4 project did not anticipate what they would culminate in.

This is probably not the line of questioning, at all.

The better line of questioning might be something like this:

"In the long run, can you really be surprised when both the 'experts' and the great mass of people believe that that Man is just lately emerged from pond scum, and we are doing the right thing when we put people out of their misery?"

While no one puts it quite like that, I can assure you, from my own research, that there are a large number of 'experts' who believe it, and the 'great mass of people' is not far behind them.

You've been warned.

Anthony Horvath

---

[8] I say 'If' as if it has not already happened again. A case can be made that it has already happened again, perhaps several times. For example, what about Rwanda?

PREFACE

This book began as an attempt on my part to gain an insight into certain missing or obscure chapters in the history of our country.

Much has already been written, both here and abroad, many attempts made to identity the motives, but I have always felt that the whole story has never been told.

As my inquiries and researches advanced, I began to realise that I had stumbled on something more significant than originally thought.

Germany had not only victimised (and I will not attempt to absolve my country) but had itself become a victim of something far more dangerous and far-reaching than National Socialism, racialism or any other 'ism.' Its foundations were laid in the early 20th century culminating during the period that Hitler set Europe ablaze and it used the insanity of war to disguise much of its activities.

The post-war reforms served as a new cover, and the kernel of a fresh social onslaught lies waiting in several countries today. I discovered that the events in Germany were the background to a few notable facts concerning the 60s and 70s.

It was at this point that I was forced to make a difficult decision. Obviously I had to make the story known to others to warn them, but should I wait until my research was complete (I had no way of knowing how much longer this might take) or should I now publish the facts I had so far collected?

I decided on the latter course. But more work needs to be done, more evidence must be collected, and more must be written. Having revealed part of the truth I hope others will wish to find out more and make their findings known.

CHAPTER I

SURPLUS PEOPLE

The basic reasoning behind the state of mind we are about to see in action has its origins in the theories of Malthus, Darwin and Galton and the development of their ideas by their "scientific" disciples.

Malthus

Thomas Robert Malthus (1766-1834) was an English political economist and historian who in 1798 published a book called *An Essay on the Principle of Population.*" This document started a reaction against the earlier writings of Godwin, Condorcet and others, who reinforced the principles of emancipation and enlightenment which ensued after the French Revolution. Malthus' theories put forward here and in later works have a surprising influence even today.

He proposed that poverty, and thereby also vice and misery, are unavoidable because population growth will always exceed food production. The checks on population growth were wars, famine, and diseases. Malthus proposed "sexual abstinence" for the working class as a means by which the population excess could be diminished and a balance achieved. In this way, the "lower" social classes were made totally responsible for social misery.

This solution was based on the hypothesis that population increased in geometric progression (2, 4, 8, 16, 32, 64, 128 and so on) while food production increased in arithmetic progression (1, 2, 3, 4, 5, 6, 7, 8 and so on). The situation already existing in his time would get worse, according to his claims and would reach alarming proportions. His basic idea can be shown pictorially in the following diagram.

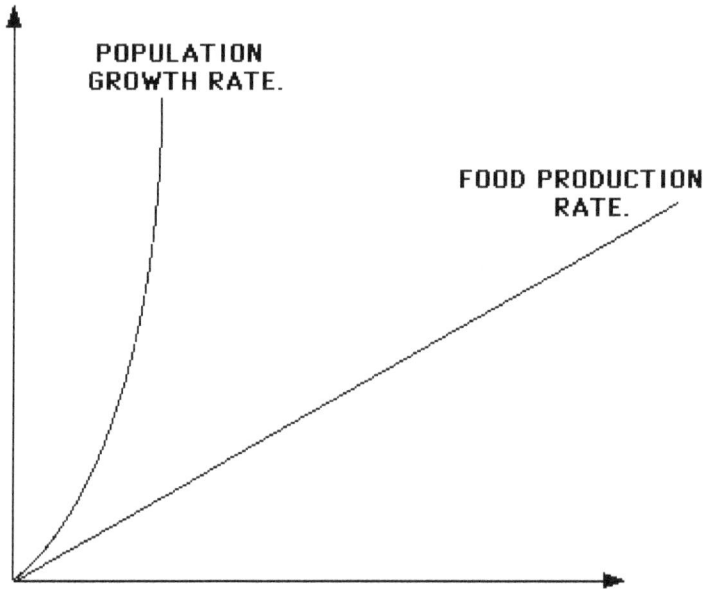

POPULATION GROWTH RATE.

FOOD PRODUCTION RATE.

Malthus was one of the earliest, but not the last, to turn away from the economic solutions of that period, and seek to solve social problems, such as poverty, through the use of biological measures. His premises, presented as facts and his figures with an air of mathematical authority, were impressive and convincing, although his ideas were based solely on some small travels and minor observations. However, despite the grand display and presentation, some of his critics realized the absurdity of it all. Both of the growth-rates were arbitrary, for there were no statistics on population increase or food production, before or during this time, which would have permitted a forecast for the future. Apart from this, no one knew just how much land was actually cultivated or partially cultivated and how much was barren

Malthus' presentations had the impact of a bomb; his mathematical and geometrical explanations and diagrams had a hypnotic effect, and only a few asked on what his claims were actually based. His theory has retained its persuasive power to such an extent that many of our present authorities use it as a basis of operation. Yet neither Malthus nor his later disciples ever managed to put forward any scientific proof for his theory, and in fact excellent scientists have at various times disproven Malthus' theory and the ideology resulting from it.

However, with the book, Malthus created an atmosphere which not only prevented a real solution to the social problems, but also promoted the repressive legislation which worsened the conditions of the poor in England. It was reasoned that better conditions for the poor would only encourage them to further propagate, putting those who were capable of work at a disadvantage. Malthusianism then moved forward to achieve its greatest triumph in 1834 with a new law providing for the institution of workhouses for the poor, in which the sexes were strictly separated to curb the otherwise inevitable over-breeding. This type of thinking has an inherent devaluation of human life through fear that the ever increasing population of lower classes will devour the more civilized or "better" people. This kind of philosophy, of course, urged the calling forth of drastic measures to handle the problem. The first resurgence took place a hundred and fifty years after his death, resulting in the birth-control movement, a principle which is based on Malthusianism. Following the Second World War, the idea was again taken up and today receives new momentum in the "population explosion" campaigns.

Darwin

Charles Robert Darwin [1809-1882], English naturalist. After years of research work formulated in 1859 his theory of evolution in his book, *The Origin of Species by Means of Natural Selection or The Preservation of Favoured Race In the Struggle for Life.* Without at that time going into a study of mankind, he tried to explain the development of life-forms in terms of a struggle for existence. The result of this struggle would be a natural selection of those species and races who were to triumph over those weaker ones who would perish.

During his research he came across Malthus' essay and suddenly saw that his own theory could be expanded to include all life in the struggle for existence that would be inevitable if food production was to lag behind the growth-rate of the population. And so Darwin took over the false doctrine of Malthus and made it a cornerstone of his own theory. In 1871 he published his next large work entitled, *The Descent of Man and Selection in Relation to Sex,* which was based on his earlier book but which dealt almost exclusively with man. In it he came to the reasonable conclusion that both in physical structure and physiological behavior, there was no difference between man and other mammals. However, the idea that this was also applicable to mental and moral qualities, shows that he was on unsound ground. Although Darwin was an excellent naturalist, he was not a very good philosopher. In his attempt to explain the social development of Man as a struggle for existence and selection through natural means, he compounded the error that Malthus had made by yet another attempt to apply a biological solution to philosophical and social problems. Darwin's speculations, to be found in his "Notebook", that thought was a brain secretion, is completely without basis.

Modern theories of evolution finally succeeded in clarifying this confusion by separating the development of man into two different steps, animal and psycho-social. Despite this, Darwin's theses and those of his followers have been very influential over a long period. They caused a significant shift in the social thinking of that time, the consequences of which can still be felt today.

Galton

Francis Galton [1822-1911] was an English psychologist and a half-cousin of Darwin. Very erratic in his thought processes, he was unable to complete research in even one area. Hardly would he begin a research project before throwing out a theory and then move on to a new field leaving the proof of the theory to others. He was so fascinated with Darwin's theory, that he spent an unusually lengthy period of years trying to prove that mental abilities were hereditary. In 1869 he published his book, *Hereditary Genius*, and in 1883, *Enquiries into Human Faculty*. In his *Enquiries* he undertook to transfer his hereditary theories from the individual to the whole race.

Galton extended Darwin's theory of natural selection into a concept of deliberate social intervention, which he held to be the logical application of evolution to the human race. Galton was by no means satisfied to let evolution take its course freely. Having decided to improve the human race through selective breeding, brought about through social intervention, he developed a subject which he called "Eugenics", the principle of which was that by encouraging better human stock to breed and discouraging the reproduction of less desirable stock, the whole race could be improved.

Social Darwinism

The pseudo-science resulting from the fusion of Darwin's evolutionary theory with social and political theories.

Charles Darwin was a very humane man, who probably would have been greatly enraged at the extremes to which his theories were taken. He had made a tragic error in attempting to extend the biological law of the struggle for survival to the social life of man. In so doing he played into the hands of "experts" of later generations, by giving them the impressive scientific justification for their barbaric actions of "natural selection," "preservation of favored races" and the "struggle for life." It was passages of the following type in *The Descent of Man* that would have been most welcomed by them:

> With savages, the weak in body or mind are soon eliminated; and those that survive commonly exhibit a vigorous state of health. We civilized men, on the other hand, do our utmost to check the process of elimination; we build asylums for the imbecile, the maimed, and the sick; we institute poor-laws; and our medical men exert their utmost skill to save the life of every one to the last moment. There is reason to believe that vaccination has preserved thousands, who from a weak constitution would formerly have succumbed to small-pox. Thus the weak members of civilized societies propagate their kind. No one who has attended to the breeding of domestic animals will doubt that this must be highly injurious to the race of man. It is surprising how soon a want of care, or care wrongly directed, leads to the degeneration of a domestic race; but excepting in the case of man himself, hardly any one is so ignorant as to allow his worst animals to breed.

Social theories based on the "survival of the fittest" had been circulating before the publication of *Origin of Species*, and even before Darwin himself. Herbert Spencer, a social theorist and scientist had already propounded the social implications of this theory some years before the appearance of Darwin's book:

> The well-being of existing humanity, and the unfolding of it into this ultimate perfection, are both secured by the same beneficent, though severe discipline, to which the animate creation at large is subject; a discipline which is pitiless in the working out of good; a felicity- pursuing law which never swerves for the avoidance of partial and

temporary suffering. The poverty of the incapable, the distresses that come upon the imprudent, the starvation of the idle, and those shoulderings aside of the weak by the strong... are the decrees of a large far-seeing providence...

or, in plain language, the fittest survive. In a later edition of *Origin of Species*, Darwin himself described Spencer's "survival of the fittest" phrase as being more accurate than his own "natural selection." Finally, in Darwin's work the social theorists had found the scientific rationale that lent respectability to their arguments. This fusion came to be known as Social Darwinism, a movement that gained increasing momentum with its demands for social legislation in accordance with the principle of "the fittest must survive," and its effects were calamitous for later generations.

Racism and Racial Hygiene

Although the beginnings of racism lie far back in history, its actual modern development really begins with the Frenchman, Arthur Count de Gobineau [1816-1882] who published his classic racist pronouncement *Essay on the Inequality of Human Races* in 1853-1857. Greatly misinterpreted by others, he wrote in a romantic fashion of a fair-haired Aryan race that was superior to all others. Gobineau maintained that remnants of this race could be found in various countries in Europe constituting a tiny racial aristocracy decaying under the overwhelming weight of inferior races. He made no special claims for the superiority of German Aryans, nor markedly denigrated other races. His racialism embraced not so much the races as the classes, the aristocracy versus the proletariat. Nevertheless, his ideas were widely distorted to fit the racial superiority theories of others. Hardly noticed in his own country, he enjoyed great popularity in Germany.

As we have already seen, an amalgamation of ideas occurred shortly before the turn of the century. Darwinism, united with social theories, became Social Darwinism, which in turn included Eugenics. In 1890, Gobineau's book was revived and in 1894 the Gobineau Association was founded in Germany. His writings were popularised at this time by the Pan-Germans, an extremely nationalistic and anti-Jewish group who, though small in numbers, were very strong, their members including a high proportion of teachers.

In 1899, Gobineau's disciples Houston Stewart Chamberlain [1855-1927], an Englishman holding German citizenship, published his two volume work, *The Foundations of the Nineteenth Century*, in Germany. It proved immensely popular and ran into many editions. Departing from Gobineau's rather flowery ideas, he upheld the German race to be the purest form of Aryanism and damned the inferior races, the Jews and Negroes, as degenerate.

Chamberlain combined the scientific fact of the existence of different races with an enriched mystical significance attached to one race, the Aryans, who had supposedly existed since the dawn of time. These mystical Aryans were held to be responsible for all the great cultures of the past, each of which had declined because the Aryans allowed other races to intermix with them resulting in the fall of that civilization—Egypt, Greece, Rome all perished.

Eugenics, Social Darwinism and Racial Hygiene now join hands, although Eugenics is the only one of these that one could manage to call a science. It is a movement which has attracted many medical men, and these have given the scientific means of assisting Social Darwinism in its endeavours to favour the fittest, and Racial Hygienists in their efforts to improve the race.

From this point on, Eugenics, Social Darwinism and Racial Hygiene fused so strongly that it would prove a useless endeavour to try to differentiate between them.

CHAPTER II

THE SURVIVAL OF THE FITTEST

In 1900, the founder of racial hygiene in Germany, Dr. Alfred Ploetz, participated in an essay contest. It was sponsored by the industrialist Alfred Krupp, who gave a prize for the best essay on the subject "What can we learn from the principles of Darwinism for application to Inner Political development and the laws of the state?"

Many people entered, and most essays agreed that a biological blue-print and a group of biologically fit must maintain a pure strain to ensure the further existence of the state.

Wilhelm Schallmeyer, who won first prize, interpreted culture society, morality, and even "right" and "wrong" in terms of the struggle for survival. He wanted all laws brought into line with these concepts to prevent the white races from degenerating to the level of the Australian Aborigines. Such a degradation would be unavoidable if society continued to pander to the physically or mentally weak. His colleague, Dr. Alfred Ploetz, endorsed the whole essay and supported the superiority of the Caucasian race from which, of course he excepted the Jews' while the Aryans were claimed as the apex of racial perfection. For instance, he suggested that in times of war in order to preserve the race, only racially inferior persons should be sent to the front. As the soldiers in the front lines are usually the ones who are killed, this would preserve the purer part of the race from being unnecessarily weakened. He further suggested that a panel of Doctors be present at the birth of each child to judge whether the child was fit enough to live, and, if not, kill it.

Eugenics Societies

In 1901 Galton delivered a lecture to the English Royal Anthropological Society stressing the various possibilities of improving human breeding under the present social, legal and moral conditions. In 1904 the first chair in Eugenics and working society in Eugenics were instituted at University College, London, and these led to the establishment of the Galton Laboratory of National

Eugenics in 1907. Soon Eugenics groups began to spring up all around the world.

In 1908 the Eugenics Education Society (renamed the Eugenics Society in the 20's) was founded in England and in 1910 the Eugenic Record Office in the United States. Both institutes used the research results of the Galton Laboratory of National Eugenics to propose practical applications, and they made it their task to intensely propagandize the eugenic idea to the public.

Dr. Alfred Ploetz, the same man who had assisted Schallmeyer with his prize essay, in 1905 founded the "Gesellschaft für Rassenhygiene" [Society for Racial Hygiene] in Germany. Later it changed its name to "Gesellschaft für Rassenhygiene (Eugenik)", which means the Society for Racial Hygiene (Eugenics). This change of name took place after Galton's announcement that racial hygiene and eugenics were in fact synonymous terms. These terms used in the German language were not only interchangeable, but racial hygiene was taken to be the German translation of eugenics. As racial hygiene was closely connected with political anthropology — a pseudo-science developed by Gobineau — eugenics was used as the scientific basis upon which racialist and political ideas, especially those of the Nazis, were based.

In 1904 Dr. Alfred Ploetz founded the journal "Archiv für Rassen-und Gesellschaftsbiologie" [Archive for Racial and Social Biology] which after one year of existence became the official organ of the "Gesellschaft für Rassenhygiene" [Society for Racial Hygiene], which Ploetz had created. A co-founder of this society was the later world-famous psychiatrist and racial hygienist, Professor Dr. Ernst Rüdin.

Eugenics Becomes a Mental Therapy

Psychiatry already had a strong physical, biological and organic foundation by this period. Emil Kraepelin, a pupil of Wundt, had earlier and in agreement with contemporaries suggested that mental and physical illnesses could be divided into two categories, those which are hereditarily caused and those due to the environment.

Psychiatrists Dr. Benedict Morel, Wilhelm Griesinger, Emil Kraepelin and Henry Maudsley in the 19th century had stressed the hereditary, biological and organic causes of mental illnesses. Their "scientific" principles had considerable influence on psychiatry and are found echoed throughout the psychiatric texts of the nineteenth century.

With the beginning of the 20th century the more brutal forms of psychiatric treatment had begun to be abandoned. The whirling stools, head-beating machines, whips, clubs and similar instruments had not proven successful, as so far no one had been healed. As more and more methods of treatment were being discarded, the profession suddenly became aware that no adequate treatment could be found to justify the existence of psychiatry as a profession. Who first had the brilliant idea is lost in the untraceable annals of endless psychiatric journals and texts, but the whole discipline gradually turned to the subject of heredity, as well as eugenics, as a possible method of eliminating mental illness even if mental illness could not be cured.

Various principles developed from an attempt to prevent further mental illness, some championed by one group, others by another, but all of them attempts to solve the problem of mental illnesses while maintaining the facade of scientific theory and practice.

"The mentally ill should not breed with non-mentally ill." This slogan led to the establishment of colonies which separated the insane and mentally defective from the rest of society.

The supporters of eugenics also believed that the result of procreation of a mentally-ill person with a mentally healthy person would be mentally-ill offspring. If the offspring were not mentally ill, the danger of a recessive gene causing a mental defect in later generations was a much too serious a danger to be tolerated.

"The mentally-ill element in the population is increasing." This slogan led to measures which were directly intended to inhibit the birth of mentally ill children. This led to a series of principles, escalating in the force of their application: separation from society, restraint, separation of the sexes in defective colonies, and sterilizations.

Mental Hygiene

Clifford Beers, a former mental patient, campaigned heavily in America for better treatment of the mentally ill. A Swiss-German professor operating in America, Adolf Meyer, coined the term "Mental Hygiene".

In 1908 the Connecticut Society for Mental Hygiene, the starting point of the Mental Hygiene movement as an organized body, was founded. Its aims were: improved treatment for the insane, and the safeguarding of the public's mental health.

In the 1920's groups were formed in other countries-Canada, France, Belgium, England, Bulgaria, Denmark, Hungary, Czechoslovakia, Italy, Russia, Germany, Austria, Switzerland, Australia. By 1930 twenty-four countries had Mental Hygiene Associations.

Routinely, these associations had as their medical specialists psychiatrists who espoused eugenic medicine and lay members who were simultaneously active in the Eugenics Societies which had by this time become very numerous.

In France, one of the leaders of mental hygiene was Dr. Edouard Toulouse, in Great Britain it was Miss Evelyn Fox, Secretary of the Central Association for Mental Welfare. She had been an active member of the Eugenics Society before the foundation of the National Council for Mental Hygiene, of which she was an officer and founder, and finally was recognized as leader of the Mental Hygiene movement as a whole. Among the board members of the National Council for Mental Hygiene was Sir Cyril Burt, who had been a member of the Eugenics Society for eleven years before the foundation of the National Council. Later he was founder of MENSA, a high I.Q. group which espouses eugenic principles. From the annual reports of the National Council for Mental Hygiene one can see many names that are also common in the Eugenics Society, including:

Dr. E. Mapother — active Eugenicist
Major Leonard Darwin — Officer of the Eugenics Society
Dr. A. F. Tredgold — Psychiatric Member of the Eugenics Society
Dr. Adolf Meyer — Member of the Eugenics Society.

The Mental Hygiene movement drew strongly from the Eugenic movements of whatever country they were in, and in fact the Mental Hygiene Movements were permeated with Eugenic thought. In 1931 the publishing firm Walter de Gruyter and Co. published the "Handwörterbuch der Psychischen Hygiene und der Psychiatrischen Fürsorge" [Handbook of Mental Hygiene and Psychiatric Care] as an official psychiatric reference work containing a high proportion of eugenically-oriented contributors. Frequent references are made throughout the book to Eugenics, Planned Marriages, Heredity,

Degeneration, etc. and under the heading "mental hygiene" we find the following:

> Therefore the hereditary constitution of a personality is the first and most effective point of prophylactic intervention: in the sense of eugenic psychiatry it is necessary to hinder unfavourable hereditary combinations and bring about favourable ones, and especially to prevent the propagation of the hereditary traits of physical illness and the socially inferior psychopathies.

The principle that prevention of birth of the mentally-ill would eradicate mental illness became an operating principle for every mental hygiene group in the world.

In Germany, as in other countries, the theoreticians and practitioners of Mental Hygiene recruited mainly from eugenically oriented groups. Among them was the psychiatrist Emil Kraepelin, a close friend of Dr. Alfred Ploetz and Dr. Ernst Rüdin, Professor of Psychiatry at Munich University, co-editor with Ploetz of the "Archiv for Rassen-und Gesellschaftsbiologie" and co-founder of the Gesellschaft für Rassenhygiene (Eugenik) [Society for Racial Hygiene (Eugenics)]. In 1933 the Nazi Reichsminister of the Interior, Wilhelm Frick, nominated Rüdin as his honorary representative on the board of directors of two German racial hygiene unions. It is even more significant that Rüdin was appointed by Frick to work together with the Ministry in the reconstruction of the German race.

On the occasion of Rüdin's 65th birthday, Ploetz honoured his achievements in the Archiv für Rassen-und Gesellschaftsbiologie:

> [so] just recently he received the Goethe Medal for Art and Science from the Führer 'in recognition of his achievements in the development of German Racial Hygiene.' The Reichsminister of the Interior Dr. Frick sent him the following telegram:

>> 'To the indefatigable champion of racial hygiene and meritorious pioneer of the racial-hygienic measures of the Third Reich I send my sincerest congratulations on his 65th birthday. May you be granted many more years to continue your research for the welfare of mankind'

The Congress of German Psychiatrists, Neurologists and Internists at Wiesbaden awarded him the Heredity Medal.

Also Dr. Luxenburger, a well known racial hygienist and colleague of Rüdin's in the Genealogical Department of the Deutsche Forschungsanstalt für Psychiatrie (German Research Institute for Psychiatry) at the Kaiser-Wilhelm Institute in Munich, and Dr. W. Wlassack, racial-hygienist and exponent of the Swiss Mental Hygiene movement, both mental hygiene theorists with a racial hygienic background.

These extreme views were not, however, limited to German Psychiatrists and Racial Hygienists. In the following examples an Englishman and Swiss Frenchman are representative of this type of thinking in other nations.

The English eugenicist Karl Pearson, first Professor for Eugenics at London University, published his thoughts at the turn of the century:

> This dependence of progress on the survival of the fitter race, terribly black as it may seem to some of you, gives the struggle for existence its redeeming features; it is the fiery crucible out of which comes the finer metal. [When wars cease] mankind will no longer progress [for] there will be nothing to check the fertility of inferior stock; the relentless law of heredity will not be controlled and guided by natural selection.

and also

> History shows me one way and one way only, in which a high state of civilization has been produced, namely the struggle of race with race, and the survival of the physically and mentally fitter race. If men want to know whether the lower races of man can evolve a higher type, I fear the only course is to leave them to fight it out among themselves.

In his book *The Foundations of the Nineteenth Century*, racist Houston Stewart Chamberlain quoted the Swiss professor August Forel with great admiration and approval:

Professor August Forel, the well-known psychiatrist, has made interesting studies in the United States and the West Indian Islands, on the victory of intellectually inferior races over higher ones because of their greater virility. "Though the brain of the Negro is weaker than that of the white, yet his generative power and the predominance of his qualities in the descendants are all greater than those of the whites. The white race isolates itself (therefore) from them more and more strictly, not only in sexual but in all relations, because it has at last recognized that crossing means its own destruction." Forel shows by numerous examples how impossible it is for the Negro to assimilate our civilization more than skin-deep, and how so soon as he is left to himself he everywhere degenerates into the "most absolute primitive African savagery." (For more detail on this subject, see the interesting book of Hesketh Pritchard, *Where Black Rules White*, Hayti, 1900; any one who has been reared on phrases of the equality of mankind, etc., will shudder when he learns how matters really stand so soon as the blacks in a State get the upper hand). And Forel, who as a scientist is educated in the dogma of the one, everywhere equal, humanity, comes to the conclusion: "Even for their own good the blacks must be treated as what they are, an absolutely subordinate, inferior, lower type of men, incapable themselves of culture. That must once for all be clearly and openly stated." (See the account of his journey in Harden's *Zukunft*, February 17, 1900).

Sterilization

Eugenics had been formulated and made known by Galton in 1883. During the following years the subject was popularised and shortly after the turn of the century eugenic organisations were set up throughout the world. The movement attracted an increasing number of supporters and adherents particularly in America and Germany. And to the extent that the organisations grew, they enlarged their sphere of political influence. The legislation of various countries started to orient itself to eugenic principles and parliaments began to enact many new laws of a purely eugenic nature. Although they varied in form and execution, they all were aimed at the same objective — the mentally deficient and the mentally ill.

Laws of a general nature provided for the establishment of institutions and colonies, enabling the mentally deficient or mentally ill to be segregated from the rest of the population, thus facilitating the control and prohibition of the procreation of the insane. Two such laws were Great Britain's Mental Deficiency Act, passed in 1913 and the South African Mental Disorders Act, passed in 1916.

Other laws were much more definite and aimed directly at the sterilization of the insane. It should be noted here that the term "sterilization" in the legislation of many American States includes castration and hundreds of such emasculations have already been carried out.

An examination of the dates of this legislation in the case of America shows it to have occurred in two waves. The first one began with the passing of a sterilization law in Pennsylvania in 1905, which the Governor immediately vetoed. However, other states followed this example and had more success. This first wave reached its peak in 1913, and then declined soon after [the War probably taking attention off domestic matters to some extent], and little activity can be traced until 1920. At this point it would appear that the pure eugenically-inspired "push" exhausted itself.

However, with the growth of the mental hygiene movement [starting in 1908 in Connecticut and spreading throughout the world in the 1920's], a second more vigorous phase was entered. The Mental Health movement in each country became the primary lobbyist for the Eugenic cause, frequently doing the front-line work of the Eugenics movements and generally acting as an authoritative pressure group with the result that eugenic principles began to appear again in legislation.

Gaining momentum throughout the 20's, a second wave of enactments and amendments passed through the legislatures under the combined pressure of the interlocking eugenic and mental hygiene movements. By 1929 this had also reached its peak in America but with the added influence of the more broadly-based mental hygiene movement the surge continued throughout other parts of the world. As a result many countries had passed or were considering the passage of laws providing for compulsory and occasionally voluntary sterilization of the mentally ill or defective, alcoholic, or socially undesirable. Amongst these were Germany, Australia (various states), New Zealand, Canada (various provinces), Finland, Sweden and many of the American states. In addition

Norway, Sweden and Switzerland included castration in their measures.

In 1932 the Minister of Health in England set up a committee to look into the whole question and the findings were published in 1936. However no law was passed probably because the public after seeing first-hand the glorious achievements of a eugenically and racially based state in Nazi Germany would have raised a tremendous outcry. With no popular support and often considerable opposition at the best of times it proved more difficult to get laws passed after 1935. As the original supposed purpose of the mental hygiene movement was improved care of the mentally ill, it is strikingly odd that the first laws passed on an international basis at the instigation of the mental hygiene movement were laws to sterilize the mentally ill and prevent them from reproducing.

Euthanasia

While the whole world was being prepared by propaganda for the sterilization of the insane, the adherent of mental hygiene and eugenics were preparing their next step.

Euthanasia by definition means an easy death. It is usually understood that it should be in a painless peaceful fashion for someone who is incurable and dying. It is also known as "mercy-killing."

In 1895, Alfred Ploetz had, as we have seen, introduced Social Darwinism into Germany and founded Racial Hygiene. In his book *Fundamental Outline of Racial Hygiene* he calls for the elimination of counter-selective processes i.e. those processes which eliminate the strong and favour the weak. Amongst these he includes war and the protection of the weak and the ill. As an illustration he gives the example of a newly married couple who give birth to a weak or malformed child who would be given an easy death with a small dose of morphine by a Board of Doctors.

In 1922, Karl Binding a Jurist and Alfred Hoche a psychiatrist wrote: *The Release of the Destruction of Life Devoid of Value*. (Die Freigabe der Vernichtung lebensunwerten Lebens). They argued in favour of euthanasia that the unfortunate are a burden to themselves and society and their parting would cause no great loss, the cost of keeping these useless people was excessive and that the State could better spend the money on more productive issues. They felt that the physically and mentally defective should be painlessly eliminated and demanded the nullification of the religious and legal barriers which stood in the way. Hoche was an influential, authoritative psychiatrist and argued that the moral attitudes towards the preservation of life would soon drop away and the destruction of useless lives would become a necessity for the survival of society.

At a German medical conference in Karlsruhe in 1921, a proposal was put forward for the legalization of Euthanasia but was rejected. At a psychiatric congress in Dresden in 1922, the same motion and report that had been presented in Karlsruhe was brought up again and again rejected. At about the same time the Monist League [one of its founders was Ernst Haeckel convinced supporter of Social Darwinism] made a similar suggestion to the Reichstag again without success.

In the U.S.A., Dr. Alexis Carrel a French-American Nobel Prize winner who had been on the staff of the Rockefeller Institute since its inception, published his book, *Man the Unknown.* In 1935, its message cannot be said to have been limited to home consumption for within three years it had been translated into nine other languages.

In his last chapter, "The Remaking of Man," Carrel repeatedly looks to Eugenics as the solution to the ills of society. He suggests the removal of the mentally ill and the criminal by small euthanasia institutions which were to be equipped with suitable gases:

> There remains the unsolved problem of the immense number of defectives and criminals. They are an enormous burden for the part of the population that has remained normal. As already pointed out, gigantic sums are now required to maintain prisons and insane asylums and protect the public against gangsters and lunatics. Why do we preserve these useless and harmful beings? The abnormal prevent the development of the normal. This fact must be squarely faced. Why should society not dispose of the criminals and the insane in a more economical manner? We cannot go on trying to separate the responsible from the irresponsible, punish the guilty, spare those who although having committed a crime, are thought to be morally innocent. We are not capable of judging men. However the community must be protected against troublesome and dangerous elements. How can this be

done? Certainly not by building larger and more comfortable prisons, just as real health will not be promoted by larger and more scientific hospitals. In Germany the Government has taken energetic measures against the multiplication of inferior types, the insane and criminals. The ideal solution would be to eliminate all such individuals as soon as they proved dangerous. Criminality and insanity can be prevented only by a better knowledge of man, by eugenics, by changes in education and in social conditions. Meanwhile criminals have to be dealt with effectively. Perhaps prisons should be abolished. They could be replaced by smaller and less expensive institutions. The conditioning of petty criminals with the whip or some more scientific procedure, followed by a short stay in hospital would probably suffice to insure order. Those who have murdered, robbed while armed with automatic pistol or machine gun, kidnapped children, despoiled the poor of their savings, misled the public in important matters, should be humanely and economically disposed of in small euthanasic institutions supplied with proper gases. A similar treatment could be advantageously applied to the insane, guilty of criminal acts. Modern society should not hesitate to organise itself with reference to the normal individual. Philosophical systems and sentimental prejudices must give way before such a necessity. The development of human personality is the ultimate purpose of civilization.

CHAPTER III

THE FÜHRER APPEARS

Hitler and his life have been dealt with by various authors. I refer the reader who is interested in more information to these. It is however necessary to briefly recount some of his early history in order to better understand events which took place later.

Adolf Hitler was born on the 20th April 1889 the son of an Austrian customs official in the upper Austrian town of Braunau close to the Inn river. Various family moves resulted in the young Hitler attending a number of different schools. At one of these in Linz from 1900 to 1904 he fell under the influence of Professor Leopold Poetsch an extremely outspoken Pan-German (he supported the Pan-German movement). In addition to Poetsch several of the other teachers were strongly anti-Jewish and Hitler at this impressionable age undoubtedly absorbed their ideas and those of a Linz anti-Jewish newspaper which he began reading regularly at this time.

After leaving school he spent the next four years doing whatever he pleased spending most of his time at Linz with the occasional visit to Vienna. In early 1908 he moved to Vienna where he rented a room and made a second unsuccessful attempt to gain entry to the Vienna Academy of Art.

Before leaving Vienna in 1913, as Hitler reveals in his *Mein Kampf*, he spent much of his time in the Hofbibliothek (City Library) where he claims to have studied the history of a number of subjects particularly, and increasingly, politico-economic theories and military-political works. Because he rarely mentioned the title of anything he had read it is difficult to determine what the actual titles of the books were but there are clues to these. The similarities between Hitler's ideas and those of Gustave Le Bon (1841-1931) the French psychologist, are so striking that one can definitely draw the conclusion that he studied Le Bon's book *Psychologie des Foules* which was translated into German in 1908 under the title *Psychologie der Massen* [Psychology of the Masses] and was acquired by the Hofbibliothek in the same year.

Hitler, as we have already seen was well steeped in Pan-German literature and must have been familiar with Gobineau. Also, Dietrich Eckart, an intimate friend and early supporter, claimed in a crudely written brochure published in 1924, that amongst other works Hitler had studied the Frenchman Vacher de Lapouge's *L'Aryen Son Role Social* published in 1899. This was later translated into German in 1939 and published in Frankfurt under the title *Der Arier und seine Bedeutung für die Gemeinschaft* [The Aryan and His Role in the Community]. Lapouge seems to have had a wide field of interest. Apart from being a leading eugenicist he also found time to engage his attention with crude social Darwinism and racism. It might have almost been Hitler speaking when Lapouge stated in his book "the idea of justice... is an illusion. There is nothing but force." And "the race, the nation, is everything."

In addition to these topics Hitler was also certainly familiar with the subject of geo-politics as formulated by its English originator Sir Halford Mackinder and German exponent Karl Haushofer. Geo-politics, a relatively unknown subject, was based on the theory that the foreign policy of a country was determined by its location natural resources raw materials and opportunities rather than its political development or outlook. Karl Haushofer (1869-1946) who was later to become teacher, adviser and friend of Rudolf Hess, visited Hitler in Landsberg prison.

When Hitler left Vienna he was, as he declared later, an absolute anti-Semite, a sworn enemy of the Marxist ideology, and very Pan-German in sentiment. His view of life was strongly Social Darwinist, Society being seen as an arena in which individuals and groups were engaged in a ceaseless struggle to assert their superiority by force and cunning.

Hitler having been declared unfit by the Austrian Army moved to Munich, applied there for the German Reichswehr, and was recruited and inducted as an infantryman in August 1914. At the end of the war he returned from a military hospital to his regiment in Munich where he performed various menial tasks. In June 1919 he received political indoctrination in "national thinking" at Munich University from the Educational or Propaganda Department of a local Group Headquarters of the Bavarian Reichswehr.

During the course, his fanaticism and vehemence attracted the attention of the organisers who recruited him as a V-man (someone charged with special assignments). Shortly after this, in July, he was made a member of an Enlightenment Commando for the Lechfeld transit camp, whose duty it was to organise psycho-political instruction for the returning soldiers in anti-socialist, national thinking, while at the same time being a training ground for the Commando personnel themselves in agitation and public speaking.

In addition to his psycho-political duties he also performed the task of being a confidential agent and spy for the Group H.Q. which was keeping a careful watch on local political groups. To accomplish this, Hitler was instructed to attend meetings of the tiny German Workers Party (D.A.P.). At first he was bored with the meetings, but as he continued to attend and was enrolled as a member, his interest increased steadily, and his involvement and activities grew. At a public meeting in February 1920 he announced the twenty-five point party programme and about this time the name of the party was changed to the National Socialist German Workers Party (NSDAP) known in its more familiar form as the Nazi Party.

Released from the army in March 1920 he threw himself wholeheartedly into party activity and proceeded to make a bid for the leadership in which he was successful. In 1921, he went to Berlin in order to give a speech there to the ultra-conservative National Club, and here established the first contacts with industrialists and business circles. During the following years these increased to an ever-widening circle of supporters including Fritz Thyssen, Alfred Hugenberg (newspapers), Alfred Krupp (heavy industry), and others. There is also some evidence for the belief that Hitler visited Switzerland during the summer of 1923 in order to receive financial support.

Also in 1923, the abortive Munich Putsch, staged by Hitler, carried his name for the first time beyond the borders of Germany and earned him a short term in Landsberg prison, where with the assistance of Rudolf Hess he wrote *Mein Kampf*. As an excellent illustration of the degree of his absorption of Social Darwinism, eugenic and racial ideas it makes fascinating, if turgid, reading. Here we meet the familiar arguments of these three groups; the merciless struggle of all life forms; the victory of the strong over the weak; the ruthless disregard for the rights of others; the Jewish menace; the advocacy of techniques for breeding of superior citizens, and so on.

Upon his release from prison in December 1924 Hitler busied himself with re-asserting his control over the party. Successes followed over the next few years and, despite various setbacks and difficulties, the seizure of power came in the year 1933.

CHAPTER IV

THE SECRET SEIZURE OF POWER

Apart from the pseudo-scientific falsehoods, myths and aggrandisement of the author, Hitler's *Mein Kampf* also contains the explanation of his plan of action. Here he deals in detail with propaganda, the leadership principle (Führer prinzip), organisation of the movement and its structure, and after the seizure of power his plans for the nation. And, after leaving Landsberg prison, Hitler proceeded to lay the foundations for his shadow state.

Within the structure of the party, bureaux offices and institutions were established which closely paralleled the actual organs of the existing government. Party officers were appointed for a wide range of offices including legal policy, health and racial matters, education etc., and Nazi organisations for the professions, members of the press, teachers, doctors etc. also came into being.

In 1933, with so much preparation behind it the Nazi Party was in an excellent position to rapidly consolidate its control of power. Other groups saw the chance to extend their control and influence as well, and they too were prepared and ready. The blueprint was to hand, all that was needed was to move the programme into top gear to achieve the desired result. The magazine of the Eugenic and Racial Hygiene Society welcomed Hitler's accession to power as a major gain for them, as he was so much in accord with their own thinking.

In June of that year, at a scientific gathering dealing with eugenic problems, Wilhelm Frick (Minister of the Interior) described the number of feeble-minded and defective children born to German parents as being huge. According to him, some authorities regarded one in five of the German population as biologically unsound. These should be prevented from reproducing because their offspring were no longer desirable.

A signal victory was scored by the eugenic and mental hygiene movement on July 14, 1933, only four months after the March elections which brought the Nazis to power. Before this date it had, according to the interpretation of a majority of judges, been illegal to perform sterilization for eugenic reasons. This was now totally reversed by the passage of the "Law for the Prevention of Hereditary Disease in Posterity" or as it was better known the Sterilization Law. The chief architect of this was Professor Ernst Rüdin, Professor of Psychiatry at the Munich University, Director of the Kaiser-Wilhelm Institute for Genealogy and Demography, and of the Research Institute for Psychiatry. Rüdin was also among the German delegates to the First International Congress for Mental Hygiene which was held in Washington in 1930 and at which he urged and intensified integration of eugenics and mental hygiene.

A short time after the passing of the Sterilization Law, he published a commentary about the meaning and purpose of the Law together with the lawyer Dr. Falk Ruttke, director of the Reich's Commission for the Public Health Service of the Interior and Arthur Gütt, the Nazi population expert and head of a government department in the Reich s Ministry of the interior.

The law itself was to take effect from 5th January 1934. Very comprehensive in scope its main purpose was to cleanse the nation of impure and undesirable elements toward the realisation of the Germanic ideal.

The categories of people covered by Law were:

(1) Anyone suffering from a hereditary disease could be sterilized by means of a surgical operation if it could be expected with some certainty, according to the experiences of medical science, that his posterity would suffer from serious physical or mental hereditary disease.

(2) Persons would be considered as hereditarily diseased in the sense of this law if they suffered from any one of the following diseases:

    (i) Innate mental deficiency
    (ii) Schizophrenia
    (iii) Manic-depressive insanity
    (iv) Hereditary epilepsy
    (v) Hereditary (Huntington's) chorea
    (vi) Hereditary blindness
    (vii) Hereditary deafness
    (viii) Severe hereditary physical abnormality.

(3) Further persons could be sterilized who suffered from severe alcoholism.

The law provided for an application from the person seeking to be sterilized and if he were unfit to act or declared incapable of managing his affairs on account of mental deficiency or not yet completed his 18th year, the legal representative was entitled to apply.

Sterilization could also be applied for by the official doctor or, in the case of an inmate of a hospital sanatorium nursing home, or prison, by the head of the Institution.

A whole legal system was set up. Courts for the prevention of hereditary illnesses were instituted called "Erbgesundheitsgerichte" (Hereditary Health Courts) and attached to the existing district courts as well as the Higher Courts. Sitting on these were always one judge and two doctors (usually psychiatrists) present in court hearings of this nature. Witnesses and specialists could be called upon and the rules for civil procedure were to be normally applied.

The Act went on to order that if the Court finally decided on sterilization it should be carried out even against the person's will, provided that the application had not originated from him alone. The official doctor had to request the police to take the necessary measures. If other methods proved of no avail the application of force was permissible.

In his book *Into the Darkness - Nazi Germany Today*, Lothrop Stoddard, an American Social Darwinist, Racist and pro-Nazi had the following comments to make after a visit to Germany where he had looked into socialised health and the eugenic courts. He states that in a conversation with an earnest young man who was officially in charge of the tuberculosis section of the public health service headquarters, he was told that:

> The treatment given a tuberculosis patient is partly determined by his social worth. If he is a valuable citizen and his case is curable no expense is spared. If he is adjudged incurable he is kept comfortable of course but no special effort is made to prolong slightly an existence which will benefit neither the community nor himself. Germany can nourish only a certain amount of human life at a given time. We National Socialists are in duty bound to foster individuals of social and biological value."

Stoddard was apparently impressed by the health measures taken by the Nazis and later in the book recounts his visit to the Upper Court for Hereditary Health in Berlin-Charlottenburg. Having long been interested in the practical applications of biology and eugenics he had studied much along these lines. He made first-hand investigations whilst in Germany which included discussions with outstanding authorities on the subject. These included official spokesmen such as Frick and Darré and leading scientists Eugen Fischer, Fritz Lenz, Hans Günther and others. It was through their recommendations that he was able to sit beside the judges during a session of the Eugenic High Court of Appeals. He also quoted Professor Günther who wrote:

> The Nordic ideal becomes for us an ideal of unity. That which is common to all divisions of the German people is the Nordic strain. The question is not so much whether we men now living are more or less Nordic; the question put to us is whether we have the courage to make ready for future generations a world cleansing itself racially and eugenically.

Stoddard went on to say—

> Without attempting to appraise this highly controversial racial doctrine (regarding the Jews), it is fair to say that Nazi Germany's eugenic programme is the most ambitious and far-reaching experiment in eugenics ever attempted by any nation.

Stoddard went on to describe various aspects of Nazi eugenic population policies but before closing his survey noted the psychological aspects of these. He had found that the rulers of the Third Reich did not stop at legal and economic measures. They were aware that ideology had to be mobilised in order to completely reach their goal. So the German people were systematically propagandized for the upbuilding of what may be described as racial and eugenic consciousness.

As if the eight categories of the sterilization law, by which one had the privilege of being sterilized, had not been enough, it was decided on the 24th of November 1933 that "habitual offenders against public morals" were to be castrated. The Nazi definition of offences against public morals also included "racial pollution".

The occurrences of the following years make it evident, that the national socialist experts had far more thorough measures in mind than simple sterilization and castration as the final solution to social problems.

The Nuremberg Laws

Germany in 1933 was a unique example of the type of political climate in which a eugenic-mental hygiene movement could thrive. Economic conditions were not so markedly different from various other countries in the world but nowhere else was the political situation so conducive to the rapid and unfettered realisation of a eugenic paradise. Although the Sterilization Law marked a major victory in the establishment of a mentally pure community, action was still needed in order to ensure racial purity. This came in 1935 with the so-called "Nuremberg Laws".

Prior to 1933 anti-Jewish acts by the Nazis had no legal basis under the Constitution. After the seizure of power a stream of anti-Jewish legislation commenced. Initially these were concerned with compulsory retirement of "non-Aryan" government employees, attempts to define "non-Aryan", and questionnaires to civil servants for details of their racial background. Also during this period "spontaneous" harassment of the Jews continued but this was largely disapproved of by the Party leaders who preferred to solve the question legally. Even Julius Streicher, the notorious and obscene Jew-baiter, publicly condemned the use of non-legal methods going so far as to accuse the perpetrators of being Jews themselves!

The climax of the initial steps was reached in the Nuremberg Party Day celebrations on September 15th 1935 when Goering, to the acclaim of the assembled Nazi officials, read out what have become known as the "Nuremberg Laws." Already preceded by an assortment of citizenship laws beginning in 1933, the two new laws were sharply to the point. The first, the Reich Law of Citizenship, divided the German nation into classes of citizens, those who were merely subjects of the State and those who possessed full citizenship including political rights. Based on racial and ideological grounds this law, with one stroke, placed all Jews into the category of second-class citizens.

The law "For the Protection of German Blood and German Honour" [the second of the Nuremberg laws and called the "Blood Protection Law" for short] was intended to ensure the racial purity of the nation for all time. Fundamentally it made criminal any sexual intercourse between both these new groups the "Reich Citizens" and the "Subjects" but it was aimed specifically at the Jews. Apart from that, this law also served as a basis for further isolation of the socially undesirable in the following years.

It goes without saying that Ernst Rüdin unblushingly claimed for the German Racial Hygiene and Eugenic Movement a measure of responsibility for the inspiration of these Laws. The aim of racial hygiene was to create a fictitious Aryan race. In accordance with this all "non-Aryan" elements had to be rooted out. Apart from having a wrong combination of chromosomes, it also seems to have been a "non-Aryan" trait to have or to be of a different opinion. Consequently, all minorities fell into this category, and liquidation, with the exception of the Jews who were declared scapegoats, started with the smallest groups and worked up from there. Because of this, the larger minorities were left with the belief that it never would be their turn. If the Nazis had started from the other end, everyone would have known that it was to be everyone's neck and they could have united themselves against this procedure when the Nazis were not yet firmly established.

Amongst the minorities that were considered "non-Aryan" were included the Gypsies, Free-masons, Jehovah's Witnesses, Jews and Christians. A common denominator of these religions and ideological minorities is that they all strongly believed in something spiritual and mental and oriented their lives according to this belief. They were unlikely to respond to a psychiatric dream-world and therefore found no place in the psychiatric view of life.

CHAPTER V

USELESS BREAD-GOBBLERS
(SS Slang)

If we look back at the numerous paths the various currents of activity took in the first three decades of the twentieth century, we see that in the Thirties they gradually amalgamated and a trend emerged in a certain direction [sterilization of the mentally ill, Nuremberg Laws etc.] which was striving to "even greater heights." The German racial and mental hygienists had prepared the ground for an all-embracing project which they called the "Euthanasia Programme," but would more accurately have been called "Mass murder of mental patients".

In 1921 the Professors Dr. Erwin Baur, Dr. Eugen Fischer, and Dr. Fritz Lenz jointly published the first edition of their two volume book, *Human Hereditary Teaching and Racial Hygiene,* which was internationally recognized as a standard text-book and soon was even used in universities abroad.

In the second volume by Dr. Lenz, first Professor for racial hygiene in Germany (the chair was established in 1923 at the Munich University), entitled *Human Selection and Racial Hygiene* (Eugenics), he wrote:

> A real restoration to health of the race cannot be begun without generous measures and the organisation of social-racial hygiene; but these are mostly only introduced when the racial hygienic idea has become the popular knowledge of the population or at least of the mental leaders. These must first develop a feeling for the senselessness of a civilization which allows the race to decay, an order of society and economics which has no regard for the interests of eternal life, which in fact is often detrimental. The introduction of racial hygienic education in the secondary schools (high-schools) and universities could effectively counter this illiteracy (lack of education); unfortunately this will only be possible when the

importance of racial hygiene has become known in the right places. As long as this is not the case, the most important practical duty of racial hygiene is the private promulgation of racial hygienic ideas. As soon as racial hygienic conviction has become a living ideology, then the racial hygienic organisation of life, even public life, will happen by itself... Anyone who loves his race cannot wish for it to fall into decadence. He must realise that the industriousness of the race is the first and unrelenting condition for the thriving of the race. Even the fight for freedom and self-assertion of the race must in the final instance serve the race. When in a fight for power the best blood is sacrificed without substituting it then it is senseless... And when racial damage has been caused through war, be it through error or because it was inevitable, it must be the first concern of those who do not want to see the race blind but seeing, to even out these damages. This is not just the substitution in number, much more important is the substitution of racial fitness. Even this requires the spirit of sacrifice and fortunately there is no lack of this — there is only a lack of understanding.

A brief look at the professional and ideological background of both of the authors of the first volume proves very interesting. Baur and Fischer had both worked devotedly in the Kaiser-Wilhelm Institute for Anthropology, Human Hereditary Teaching and Eugenics, in which Rüdin first acted as curator.

Baur, the biologist, later became the first Nazi Rector of Berlin University, where Fischer later lectured as a Professor for Anthropology. In his debasement of knowledge, Fischer sank to the depths of praising Hans F.K. Günther, the author of *Racial Knowledge of the German Race,* who was a popular target for general ridicule even in Germany, before the Nazis promoted him to a university professorship.

Later, in 1941, Dr. Otmar Freiherr von Verschuer, Nazi professor and former colleague of Baur, Fischer and Rüdin in the above mentioned Kaiser-Wilhelm Institute, supported the Baur-Fischer-Lenz textbook with warm recommendations.

Verschuer was the founder and first director of the Institute for Hereditary Biology and Racial Research at Frankfurt University opened in 1934. Even if it produced nothing else it brought a further star into the Nazi sky; Verschuer's former assistant Dr. Joseph Mengele. From this position he later advanced to be one of the most infamous doctors in the concentration camp at Auschwitz, where he conducted experiments with living and fully conscious prisoners and tortured the camp-inmates for the benefit of "scientific advancement." After the war, Mengele succeeded in escaping the Allies and the law, he left Germany and fled via Italy to Paraguay, settled there, acquired citizenship in his new home country and apparently lives there to this day. The time of his peaceful existence however, will hopefully soon be over; the well known Nazi criminal hunter, Wiesenthal, is on his tracks and will not rest until he has caught up with him.

At the 12th meeting of the International Federation of Eugenic Organisations, held in 1936 in Holland, Verschuer appeared as the representative of his Institute together with Ploetz, Rüdin and Fischer. One of the papers read to the meeting was by fellow delegate Professor Karl Astel from Himmler's SS "Race and Resettlement Office" (RuSHA).

In 1923, Lenz took a further step forward in his endeavours to find a solution to racial hygienic problems by stating that Euthanasia definitely had its place in the racial hygiene plan. The propaganda drums beat without pause, but it was only in the Thirties that the fatal Euthanasia propaganda campaign broke loose and went far beyond Germany's borders.

In July 1931 the Union of Bavarian Psychiatrists held a Congress at Munich University. V. Faltlhauser, psychiatrist and active proponent of the mental hygiene movement, who was striving towards yet greater achievement of the euthanasia programme, laid bare the basic thoughts behind the campaign for sterilization and euthanasia with the following words:

> Here we will only discuss sterilization. Basically it represents only one of the paths which lead towards the goal. You know that these measures are heavily opposed. Not only is the unjustified claim, that the question of heredity has not been clarified enough, the obstacle; the obstacles lie rather as already stated in ideological moral and ethical considerations, they lie in the idleness of the broad masses and in obsolete views which I do not wish to

go into here. This outlook must cause us to advance carefully but steadily. What primarily seems to be needed is educational work and propaganda for the broad masses, and the facts have to be constantly hammered into them. And this is also one of the many duties of our public welfare section, which should point out this fact in private life and in lectures. It will also be our imperative task to research and make more exact the laws of heredity and their final consequences. And herein again a special task will fall to our public welfare section. At this point I cannot suppress the comment that it must have other methods than those at its disposal today. Today the welfare doctors are swamped in their social tasks especially when you consider they have to do their work in a subsidiary office. If the public welfare section is to do justice to the requests for research made of it, then it should be provided with the means and the personnel. I know what I am demanding at this time of scarce means. But it must be said to prevent the blame being put on public welfare, as it has failed to fulfill demands put on it.

When demanding sterilization, compulsory action is at present to be avoided; on the other hand voluntary sterilization is to be promoted by any means. For this a clear unequivocal legal safety precaution must be created. It is quite evident that even voluntary sterilization must be based on certain prerequisites and safety precautions and that clear, flawless, medically-determined indicators must be present. What these safety precautions are to look like, whether it is to be a commission or not, whether the commission should consist of doctors, civil-servant doctors or be mixed etc. is a question to be considered and is not relevant to the principle. The clear indication will be in the cases of the gravest strain, which with today's knowledge we must now recognize will have a high probability of heavy hereditary defects in the descendants. It need only be mentioned incidentally that sterilization is only to occur in the form of severing the spermatic duct whilst preserving the gonads or the operative interruption of the Fallopian tube. Also the question of possibly demanding compulsory sterilization in the cases of criminal tendencies and high-probability hereditary insanity should also be considered. This however should occur only when the broad masses have intensively been worked over in the ways mentioned earlier, and have become mature enough to accept such ideas.

Many have said that internment is the only sound measure against the bearers of very bad hereditary mass. But quite apart from the fact that it is the most expensive preventive measure, is it really more humane and a lesser violation of the principle of personal freedom? Do we not forcibly prohibit the party concerned from procreation for their whole life?

We Germans cannot totally neglect events which occur outside our borders. A whole series of nations have positively accepted that the laws of heredity do affect the development of mental abnormality and have understood the consequences of that and created sterilization laws. The Americans have been reproached with reckless pluck because of laws they have passed in 22 of their states. But when we see that an otherwise cool and calculating race such as the Danes pass a sterilization law, how the canton Waadt has also done this, when the Swedish ministries are seriously dealing with this problem, then this must really give us something to think about.

Before I end, I must permit myself a few short comments which are forced upon me by an objective conscience. I believe that we must beware of exaggerated expectations of the success of sterilization. Sterilization, even compulsory, will not be able to plug all the fountains of bad hereditary mass.

The principle used here to hoodwink the public into accepting enforced sterilization is to first start a propaganda campaign for voluntary sterilization. This same rule also applies for compulsory euthanasia where propaganda starts with the introduction of voluntary euthanasia. Both Germany and England were literally flooded with Euthanasia campaigns.

In England, Dr. Charles Killick Millard, President of the Society of Medical Officers of Health, brought up in his 1931 Presidential speech the question of voluntary euthanasia and proposed a suitable law. A few years later, he became a fellow founder of the Voluntary Euthanasia Legislation Society and its Honorary Secretary.

In 1935, Lord Moynihan, President of the Royal College of Surgeons, founded the Euthanasia Society. A year later this Society handed its recommendations for a Euthanasia project to the House of Lords. Among other things, it provided for the possibility of incurably ill persons being able to petition a Euthanasia Office of the Ministry of Health to let themselves be delivered from their sufferings. It suggested that the applicant should, after consulting his close relatives, handle his estate and choose two medical advisors and a doctor. The Ministry could give its consent for the mercy death to take place after a period of seven days, time allowed for the chance of a change of heart, or an appeal if the relatives so desired. This proposal was fortunately turned down.

However, as early as 1923, a step in this direction was taken in Switzerland and a draft for such a law was presented in Denmark in 1924. In the U.S.A., The Chamber of Doctors of the State of Illinois even requested the approval of mercy death. The year 1938 was marked by the establishment of the American Society of Euthanasia, and on similar lines, a society for voluntary euthanasia was founded in Connecticut and drafts of laws were presented to the parliaments of Nebraska and Canada in 1937. In Germany, the activities in the field of euthanasia, reached their climax. In 1934, Baur, who had long advocated the sterilization law, foretold that such a law would only be a start.

The actual campaign for euthanasia in Germany took many forms. Films were produced (among others "I accuse") which were to make obvious that there were useful and less useful members of society, and were intended to cause astonishment on the part of the viewer as to why anybody bothered to prolong these unproductive human lives at all. Articles in newspapers informed the reader about costs caused by the mentally ill and showed plainly how the money could be used for more productive and creative things. The campaign was so extensive that it even reached school books, in which the nature of the problems were to direct the attention of the pupil to this subject. One such example is the arithmetic textbook written in 1935 by Alfred Dorner, whose series of distorted and disguised questions were to have the desired influence.

So we see that sterilization and euthanasia were not the ideas of the Nazis and never had been. They were ideas which were supported and promoted throughout the whole world by groups with a strong interest in the progressive development of mental hygiene and mental health. There is no doubt that euthanasia was supported in many countries, among them America, Finland, England, Denmark, Sweden, Norway, Australia and New Zealand. Germany however was the only country in which the political climate was such as to allow materialization of the final goal of the supporters of sterilization and euthanasia.

Sterilization laws at the same time were preparing the ground in other countries such as U.S.A. (some states) for much larger endeavours. However the step from sterilization to murder is great (though apparently less great for someone who has fully absorbed the state of mind of the mental hygiene movement). Therefore it seems only logical that one tried to win the politicians to the new ideals, to manipulate them and to appoint them in the right places, in order to bring about the desired goal. In Germany the politicians were ideal for this purpose, and consequently the action moved much faster there. But, as we will see later, because of the German activities, the attitude towards the subjects of sterilization and euthanasia changed shortly after the Second World War.

The next step, towards the end of 1938 and the beginning of 1939, was publicly tested in Germany after endless discussions and propaganda moves. A letter addressed to Adolf Hitler written by a man called Knauer from Leipzig asked for permission for a doctor to shorten the fife of his child who was born blind, seemed to be an idiot and had only parts of its arms and legs. The child itself was at this time at the Children's Clinic in the University of Leipzig, which was headed by Professor Werner Catel, Professor for Neurology and Psychiatry at the same university.

At that time Catel was already an exponent of euthanasia and has remained one to this day, which fact he acknowledged in his book *Border Situations of Life - Contribution to the Problem of a Limited Euthanasia*. It was Catel who made the suggestion to the father, or at least focused his attention in that direction, to write a letter to the Führer. As an answer to this letter, Hitler sent his physician, Professor Karl Brandt, to Leipzig and after consultations with Catel, put the child to sleep.

Several months later, Hitler signed a document authorizing Dr. Karl Brandt and Reich-leader Philipp Bouhler to permit euthanasia in special cases. This authorization was supposedly signed in October

1939, but was backdated to the beginning of September of the same year. The document was really nothing more than an authorization and formulated in such a way that a doctor who truly felt bound to the Hippocratic Oath could interpret it in such a way that no-one would have to die. The "Führer-order" as it was generally called, had apparently come about after a lively discussion between Dr. Karl Brandt, Dr. Leonardo Conti and Philipp Bouhler and was as follows:

> Reichsleader Bouhler and Dr. Brandt M.D. are charged with the responsibility of enlarging the authority of certain physicians to be designated by name in such a manner that persons who according to human judgement can upon most careful diagnosis of their condition of sickness be accorded a mercy death.

Signed — A. Hitler.

In spite of this, the document was regarded not only as a "legal" basis for the crimes committed by the psychiatrists of Nazi Germany, but later at the Nuremberg trials and in other court cases, it was used as a justification where the accused attempted to interpret this authorization as an order.

The question about the so-called "Führer-order" is usually done away with by stating that Hitler wanted to achieve one of his goals with this document. However, several facts contradicted this widespread theory and should be mentioned in this context. Obviously Hitler agreed or at least sympathized with the arguments of the eugenically-oriented groups, which were trying to defend sterilization and euthanasia. This we know from his earlier studies and activities, but one cannot charge him with having voiced his opinion in this direction very often. On the contrary, he seldom remarked on it. The actual document was very vague, and it is not even clear that the victims were to be hopelessly mentally ill, but only referred to incurably sick generally. The previously mentioned Knauer case is a typical example of the psychiatric way of thinking and their tactics.

The Third Reich is usually looked upon as a monolithic state, a pyramid structure with Hitler at the top followed by the administrative machinery of government and its subordinate organisations, which form a wide basis, the whole system unified and dynamic. In actual fact, the Third Reich was a system of agencies, departments and branches of government all in competition with each other. All endeavoured to play each other off against each other for reasons of prestige, in order to win the favour of the Führer or to increase their power. Hitler himself issued different versions of the same order to keep his subordinates divided and in competition with each other. This way there was less chance of their becoming dangerous to him.

Hitler had purposely disarranged the "whole" structure of the Reich, with the aim of achieving a shift of emphasis of function, a tactic which proved successful in ensuring his own position of power. Apart from the actual government offices the NSDAP committees established before the seizure of power remained in existence, so that Hitler had two organisations at his disposal with greatly overlapping functions. The administration of the Third Reich was, therefore, a chaotic confusion of conflicts, jealousies and duplication of actions. An order which was not taken up by someone and worked on or passed on just remained an order, and ended up in a desk-drawer, never executed. Actually a great deal of effort was necessary to get a lot of things moving at all.

Additionally, after the seizure of power, Hitler was only interested in activities for which he had a special affinity and he neglected other activities. Ministers and functionaries often did not see him at all for long periods of time. To the degree that Hitler engrossed himself in the plans for the expansion of the Reich, he had to deal more and more with the solution of military problems and with diplomatic matters. His interest in non-military matters and initiatives declined

Thus because Hitler's attention was unequivocally on other matters, the "experts" who were continuously exerting pressure on internal affairs, such as initiating the mass-murder of mental patients, also assumed responsibility for it. This is affirmed by the two well known and informed American journalists William L. Shirer and Joseph Harsch both active as foreign correspondents in Berlin in those years.

Shirer collected his impressions in his "Berlin Diary" published in England in 1941. Towards the end of his diary notes the author deals with his experiences with the euthanasia programme. He writes:

What is still unclear to me is the motive for these murders. Germans themselves advance three:

1. That they are being carried out to save food.

2. That they are done for the purpose of experimenting with new poison gases and death rays.

3. That they are simply the result of the extreme Nazis deciding to carry out their eugenic and sociological ideas.

Shirer continues with his views and comes to the conclusion:

The first motive is obviously absurd, since the death of 100,000 persons will not save much food for a nation of 80 million. Besides, there is no acute food shortage in Germany. The second motive is possible, though I doubt it. Poison gases may have been used in putting these unfortunates out of the way, but if so, the experimentation was only incidental. Many Germans I have talked to think that some new gas which disfigures the body has been used, and that this is the reason why the remains of the victims have been cremated. But I can get no real evidence of this.

And now he comes to a very interesting section in which he writes:

The third motive seems the most likely to me. For years a group of radical Nazi sociologists who were instrumental in putting through the Reich's sterilization laws have pressed for a national policy of eliminating the mentally unfit. They say they have disciples among many sociologists in other lands and perhaps they have.

Paragraph two of the form letter sent the relatives plainly bears the stamp of this sociological thinking: "In view of the nature of his serious, incurable ailment, his death, which saved him from a life long institutional sojourn, is to be regarded merely as a release."

Some suggest a fourth motive. They say the Nazis calculate that for every 3 or 4 institutional cases, there must be one healthy German to look after them. This takes several thousand good Germans away from more profitable employment. If the insane are killed off, it is further argued by the Nazis, there will be plenty of hospital space for the war wounded should the war be prolonged and large casualties occur.

This information which Shirer for some reason does not consider or puts aside as being absurd or unimportant, when examined, proves to be rather useful. Of the motives the Germans propagate as their reason for these murders, three seem to hold up under examination.

The first motive, however, that they were committed to save food, originated before these measures were brought in, and thus seems quite a logical conclusion. However when one looks at the result and when one compares 100,000 patients with eighty million as Shirer had done, the whole thing stands out as absurd.

The second reason, that the murders had been committed in order to experiment with new poisonous gases, also makes sense. In the beginning stages of the euthanasia programme, many experiments were carried out to find the most effective and fastest method of exterminating the victims.

The third motive which the Germans propagated themselves, was that these murderous actions were the result of extreme National Socialists who wanted to materialize their social-hygienic and social ideas. As the whole programme was kept strictly confidential and therefore was known only by a very few people, it seems as though the Nazis had carried it out themselves. However, from the history of the preparations for these murder actions, it is obvious [and in the following chapter we will go into this in detail] that it was the extremist psychiatrists and the Nazis who together put these ideas into action.

The fourth motive offered to Shirer by some Germans, that new gases were used which deformed bodies and that this was the reason for the cremation of the mortal remains is also worth examining in more detail. The new gas, which was used in the beginning was not so new. In fact, it was simply carbon monoxide from combustion engines which did indeed deform bodies. The patients usually died under circumstances which caused deformations [some of the bodies discoloured and excrement and other fluids ran out]. It is evident that they were often in a condition which did not permit them to be put in a coffin and to be transferred. A further point which must be considered is that such a corpse, if returned to relatives would hardly have stood up to an examination to confirm the cause of death, should the family have wanted it.

The distressing thing about Shirer's Diary is that he received his information from Germans not as a rumor but as fact, and obviously obtained it first hand. He describes the Nazis as sociologists and probably uses this term as a collective term which includes psychiatrists, psychologists, anthropologists, socio-hygienists and mental hygienists. And his conclusion is correct. They were racial, they served as tools to pass the Sterilization Laws, they exerted pressure to direct the national politics towards the elimination of the mentally ill and they were very successful in all these. Shirer's claim that German sociologists had many supporters abroad was also valid.

Joseph Harsch the second American journalist in Berlin, confirms Shirer's information in his book *Pattern for Conquest*.

> Those who proposed it (the plan for euthanasia) are understood to have asked Hitler for a written edict, or law which would officially authorize them to proceed with the "mercy killings." Hitler is represented as having hesitated for several weeks. Finally, doubting that Hitler would ever sign the official order the proponents of the project, drafted a letter for him to sign which merely expressed his, Hitler's, general approval of the theory of euthanasia as a means of relieving incompetents of the burden of life. While this letter did not have the character of law it was adequate in Nazi Germany. The Führer had expressed approval of the practice. It went ahead.

Following the Knauer case, a group of competent specialists were called to the Reich Chancellery to form a Euthanasia Committee. Psychiatrist, and ministerial adviser for health in the Reich Ministry, SS Oberführer Dr. Herbert Linden, was appointed as its head. Later Linden was to act as liaison between the Chancellery and the Reich Health Service, which was attached to the Ministry of the Interior and led by Reich Doctor Führer Leonardo Conti. The founding of this committee was the first of what were to become regular meetings of the medical advisers for the purpose of better estimating the necessary administrative and technical facilities.

Lindens committee consisted of:

Professor Hans Heinze, Chief of the Brandenberg Mental Institute.
Professor Werner Catel, Lecturer in Neurology and Psychiatry at Leipzig University and head of the Paediatric Clinic in Leipzig.
Dr. Helmut Unger, Ophthalmologist, author of a novel on the euthanasia question ("Mission and Conscience") and Press liaison officer for the Reich Doctor Führer Dr. Wagner.
Dr. Ernst Wentzler Paediatrician.

Linden rapidly expanded the committee with the following additional specialists for neurology and psychiatry:

Professor Max de Crinis, Lecturer in Neurology and Psychiatry at Berlin University, secret agent and friend of Waiter Schellenburg-who held a high post in the Nazi Secret Service. [Dr. Crinis was involved in the Venlo Incident staged shortly before the outbreak of the Second World War in which two British and a Dutch Intelligence agent were kidnapped by the Germans].

Professor Berthold Kihn, Lecturer in Neurology and Psychiatry at the University of Jena.

Professor Carl Schneider, Lecturer in Neurology and Psychiatry at Heidelberg University.

Dr. Hermann Pfannmüller, who was Dr. Faltlhauser's assistant in the Asylum at Kaufbeuren and as of 1938 Director of the Mental Hospital Eglfing-Haar.

Dr. Bender — director of the Buch Mental Hospital near Berlin.

A short time later the special advisers to T4 were attached:

Professor Werner Heyde, Lecturer in Neurology and Psychiatry at Würzburg University.

Professor Paul Nitsche, Lecturer in Psychiatry at Halle University up to 1939. Director of the Sonnenstein institute near Pirna, which became one of the murder schools.

Now having the necessary advice from the "experts" about the size of the problem, of numbers, where, when, how, who, etc., the administrative machinery of T4 was put together. The programme had been drawn, the task could commence.

CHAPTER VI

THE DEATH MACHINE

The T4 Program

There is not a great deal known about T4 in comparison with other aspects of Nazi Germany and the Second World War; what little is known is difficult to verify and amongst the accounts there is conflicting or contradictory data. T4, in fact, was the Führer Chancellery and the initials "T4" came from the full address which was Tiergartenstrasse 4, Berlin. However, it is important to bear in mind two factors when attempting to appreciate the lack of information.

T4 was the source of orders and measures which were "Geheime Reichssache" [Secret Reich Matters] and those involved who served as tools in its execution were bound by silence. The euthanasia programme was considered to be one of these, and this is one of the reasons why there is so little information, with much of it conflicting, concerning its workings and its relation with the Chancellery itself. A second factor to be borne in mind is that the whole thing was planned with great care prior to the signing of the authorization by Hitler and in fact meetings involving top German psychiatrists had been taking place some months prior to the date of his authorization. As it was a very thorough programme, the creators were sufficiently foresighted to take steps to cover their tracks and conceal the evidence. One of their more brilliant ideas was to finally assign the personnel who had been trained in the euthanasia institute, and who later went on to much bigger things, to theatres of war where their survival was most certainly to be minimal. Many of the personnel were assigned to the Jugoslav front where Tito's partisans had a reputation for never taking prisoners, and a great many of them died there.

The "Project T4" was fully integrated into the organisational structure of the Reich and fell under section IIb. "Mercy-death" of the Chancellery of the Führer [KdF]. It was divided into two departments the administrative one headed by Philipp Bouhler, a shadowy figure (once described as one of the dictators of the dictators) and the medical section headed by Hitler's personal physician Dr. Karl Brandt.

In the middle of 1939 the end-phase of the administrative preparations of the euthanasia programme was started. It dealt almost entirely with keeping it secure and secret. The German people were under no circumstances to become suspicious and the project was to roll without any interference. It was therefore necessary to disguise the activities as much as possible.

Questionnaires had already been prepared by the psychiatric committee and advisers, and in October these were sent to the mental institutions of Germany. These questionnaires required answers to a number of questions including name, marital status, nationality, next of kin, whether regularly visited and by whom, who bore the financial responsibility and how long in the institution, how long sick, diagnosis, chief symptoms, whether bed-ridden, whether under restraint, whether suffering from an incurable sickness or complaint, and whether a war injury or not. And, what was the race of the patient. These questionnaires were prepared and sent out by one of the front groups which operated under T4.

In classic psychiatric style four front groups had been set up to shield the actual source of the operations in T4 from scrutiny. The idea being essentially that T4 itself would issue orders to the front group who would then carry out the necessary measures. Anybody seeking to trace back the administrative chain, say from a hospital where patients were being taken to be murdered, would arrive at one of these four front groups and the chances of getting any further back than that were very small.

The front group which sent out the questionnaires, had them returned and handled them, was named Realms Work Committee for Institutions for Cure and Care. This became the Headquarters for the whole of the organisation and was started for this purpose.

There was a parallel organisation, another front group devoted exclusively to the killing of children, for obviously some specialization was needed in this area, and the front group catered for those who had knowledge and experience of children. It was known under the ambiguous name of Realms Committee for Scientific Approach to Severe Illness due to Heredity and Constitution. In association with these two organisations were the Charitable Company for the Transport of the Sick which transported patients to the killing centers, and the Charitable Foundation for Institutional Care which was in charge of making the final arrangements.

The decree of the Reich Ministry of the Interior of August 18 1939, which introduced the requirements for registration of "deformed new-born" was a great advantage to the children project. At first this applied only the children up to the age of 3, but after 1941 this project included youths to the age of 16.

These four cover organisations safeguarded the project T4, the Reich Chancellery, and the euthanasia committee from unwanted discoveries. Those who took the initiative were very secure and if anyone had attempted to retrace the administrative chain, let us say from an institute whose patients were moved to killing-institutes, he would probably have reached one of the four cover organisations. The chances that he would get much further were very small.

Ironically the relatives of the patients were charged with the cost of the killing, without however being informed as to what they were paying for. The questionnaires having been sent out were completed by the psychiatrists, doctors in charge of the patients in the asylums. When the questionnaires came back they were evaluated by the psychiatric and professional members of T4 who were mainly leading professors of psychiatry in German Universities. The whole business was in keeping with the euthanasia programme in that no one was ever actually examined in person, in direct violation of any normal medical approach or standards, especially when one considers that life or death hung on the decision of the psychiatrist evaluating. Processing of the questionnaires was done very rapidly; for example one expert between November 14th and December 1st 1940 evaluated 2,109 of them.

At the beginning of the euthanasia programme and for some time during it, Jews were very carefully excluded from amongst the people who were being accorded a blessed release from their sufferings. The reason, apparently, was that such a worthwhile fate was obviously not to be given to Jews, that only Germans could benefit by such a humane measure. That the euthanasia programme was such a haphazard stab at resolving the social problem as an emergency measure was shown by the approach and organisation of the whole thing.

At the time the questionnaires went out, or perhaps even earlier, a number of mental hospitals or convenient buildings were being converted for their later use and were to be the killing centers and schools for murder. Death chambers were erected in the buildings disguised as shower-baths and crematoriums both of which were identical to those later to be established in the Jew-killing centers in Poland.

There appear to have been six principal death institutes and murder schools, and these were Grafeneck, Hadamar, Hartheim (in Austria), Brandenberg, Bernberg, and Sonnenstein, the hospital of the super-expert Dr. Nitsche. The system seems to have worked in the following fashion.

On the basis of the replies to the questionnaires, the Institute from which they had been returned were notified that a number of patients were to be moved, allegedly to make available beds for the war wounded, or to be moved for better treatment. A number of reasons were made known or put around as the reason for removal. These patients were collected by the front organisation Charitable Transport Company for the Sick, which then took them to one of these killing centers, where they were exterminated within a few hours of their arrival. As a further camouflage they were not always taken directly to the killing centre; on some occasions they were taken to an intermediate hospital where people were led to believe that they were there to be placed under observation.

The total number of victims of the euthanasia programme is difficult to determine but as there were 300,000 to 320,000 mental patients in 1939 and only 40,000 in 1946 it would seem that the figure of 275,000 deaths mentioned in the Nuremberg Trials was reasonably accurate.

The victims were not confined to mentally incurable patients; as the programme progressed and gained momentum other undesirables were included. It was obviously too great an opportunity to be missed to not include anyone else who wasn't worthy of life. Amongst those caught up in the dragnet for the murder institutes were psychotics, schizophrenics, patients suffering from infirmities of old age, as well as epileptics, and other patients suffering from a variety of organic neurology disorders, including the various forms of infantile paralysis, parkinsonism, multiple sclerosis and brain tumors. We also know that children were disposed of similarly, when the orphanages and reformatories were searched for further candidates.

It should be borne in mind that according to one expert at least 50% of the patients murdered would, if allowed to survive, have been able to recover and lead useful lives.

As we have seen, T4 went into a great deal planning to disguise its operations and those of the killing centers as ordinary mental hospitals and this was testified to in the Nuremberg trials by Viktor Brack, the chief of the whole section II of KdF and therefore one of the main persons responsible for the smooth execution of the euthanasia program. At the Nuremberg trials, he testified that patients walked calmly in with their towels and stood with their lithe pieces of soap under the shower outlets waiting for the water to start running.

I have been able to find more material on some murder institutions than others, but the following account could be taken as fairly representative of the other five murder institutions. Hartheim was situated near Linz which was in turn also close to Hitler's birthplace in Austria. It was an old castle dedicated as an asylum to the poor, feeble minded and stupid in 1898. Hartheim, in company with the other institutions, not only served as a murder institute for the disposal of mental patients, but also functioned as a murder school for personnel. The medical directors in charge of Hartheim were two doctors, Dr. Rudolf Lohnauer, an Austrian who later became an expert in 14f13 of which we will hear more later, and Dr. Georg Renno. They took their orders direct from T4 and were responsible for the "medical" training of personnel. The training of staff was designed to harden the personnel psychologically to the experience of having to exterminate and observe the deaths of tens of thousands of people, day after day, week after week, apart from any technical training they were given. However, from later activities in the operation of the death chambers and crematoriums, it was obvious that they were being schooled for bigger things in the workings of the Third Reich. Most of the personnel concerned in these later activities had passed through one of these murder schools.

The administrative official in charge at Hartheim was Captain Christian Wirth, a former policeman, who had been selected by T4 to supervise the training. Apart from being paid for disposing of unwanted mental patients, and to train personnel, these institutes also provided scientific testing grounds for the perfection of the murder techniques as devised by the psychiatrists on the euthanasia committees of T4. The deaths of the victims were clinically studied photographed and perfected. In the war crimes trials that took place after the war in Germany, it was proved that in the death camps of Belzec, Sobibor and Treblinka, special photographers also took pictures of people being gassed, just as they had at Hartheim and other institutes. In addition, experiments took place with various mixtures of gases in order to perfect the most effective one. During these tests, psychiatrists with stop-watches would observe the dying patients through the peepholes in the cellar door, which served as the gas chamber in Hartheim, and the length of the death struggle was clocked down to one-tenth of a second. Slow motion pictures were made and studied by the psychiatric experts at T4 in Berlin. People's brains were photographed to see exactly when death had occurred. Nothing was left to chance. The psychiatrists were very thorough.

The actual training of the students proceeded in an orderly progression of familiarisation. At first they watched the experiment as observers, as their training progressed they graduated to participation in the actual murders by conducting the patients into the chambers, releasing the gases, watching during the death struggle and finally ventilating the chambers and removing the bodies. The selection of the students was conducted by the high ranking Nazi officials who were personally and directly responsible to the Führer Chancellery.

The whole operation was shrouded in very tight security. Everybody involved realized that there could be no slip-ups — there could be no leakage of information, because they weren't dealing with sub-humans and Jews; these victims were Germans and Austrians and the reaction of the public would be very strong. And in fact, when the programme later became obvious to the inhabitants in the vicinity of the murder institutes, there was an outcry against it.

Obviously, after so much familiarity with the deaths of the victims, the students became insensible to the cries and pleas of the murdered. In the process of their being hardened, the students were observed closely by their teachers who noted their reactions and made reports on their progress as pupils. If the students were able to observe and participate in the murders of their own nationalities, even though they were deformed or mad and were of German or Austrian nationality, how much easier it would be to do the same to "sub-humans." Students who didn't complete the course because they cracked, couldn't go o in with it or were unsuitable, were sent to the war front where the Commander in charge of the unit would assign them to a suicide squad. This would account for the lack of people with conscience willing to come forward to testify to what had been involved in.

The total number of victims at Hartheim is difficult to estimate, but at the Dachau trial in 1947 testimony was given that from 30-40 unwanted humans were "treated" in the cellars *every day*. As Hartheim was in operation for about three years that would account for about 30,000 people. Hartheim also had another purpose. It served as a safety valve when executions taking place in nearby concentration camps such as Mauthausen and Dachau became more than the staff could manage. Victims were sent to Hartheim and "dispatched" there. Later, towards the end of the war Hartheim became just another place for extermination, its staff and personnel having been assigned to other duties. It was well situated for use in the euthanasia programme lying near a railway, but not too close, and around the castle were a few little houses and farms. It was 17 kilometers from Linz and from there only another 23 kilometers from Mauthausen.

Schooling of the personnel produced perfect murderers who were used to the smell of burnt flesh, had been taught how to trick people being led to their death, and how to steel themselves against the crying and pleading of the victims. Pupils were naturally rewarded, not only with alcohol and women, which were always kept handy for them, but also received medals. Usually, these were the Iron Cross Second Class and, unlike other awards which had noted in the register the reason for their being given, in these cases " Geheime Reichssache" [Secret Reich matter] was noted in the appropriate column.

One of the murder institutes, Hadamar, achieved some notoriety at the time of the euthanasia programme. In December 1939 a member of the Court of Appeals of Frankfurt-on-Main wrote to the Minister of Justice complaining about the situation. He said that among the population there were constant discussions over the question of the destruction of the socially unfit, especially in places where there were mental institutions. Vehicles used to transport the mental patients from the institutes had come to be recognized by the inhabitants. With busloads of victims converging on Hadamar, things had reached such a state that even the children were calling out as the buses passed that "they are taking some more people to be gassed."

The writer had obviously found out enough to be able to describe in his letter that there were stories circulating about transported victims being immediately stripped to the skin, dressed in paper shirts and forthwith taken to a gas chamber where they were liquidated with hydrocyanic acid gas, and the bodies reported to be moved to crematoriums by means of conveyor belts, six bodies to a furnace. He also went on to recount rumors about future victims and believed that these would include the inhabitants of Homes for the Aged and others. Interestingly, the psychiatrist in charge at Hadamar was Dr. Adolf Wahlmann an active member of the German mental hygiene movement, who had demonstrated cardiazol-shock treatment to delegates from the European Mental Hygiene Reunion (which took place in Munich in 1938).

This was not, however, the only letter of complaint, and many more followed when the never-ending smoke that fined the skies in the vicinity of the institutes for murder indicated that something was obviously terribly wrong. Various members of the communities (usually people with some standing), sent complaints to whoever they thought would be in a position to act. The main source of complaints appear to have come from the Church, and protests were raised by various Bishops and Cardinals usually addressed to the Ministry of Justice. The Bishop of Limburg for instance addressed a complaint to the Ministry concerning the institute of Hadamar, and it was very similar to the one by the member of the Court of Appeals, mentioned earlier, when children were calling out as the vans arrived, only now parents were even threatening their children that if they weren't quite bright, they would be put in the oven at Hadamar.

Obviously, with the mounting protests and complaints, the whole operation was receiving far too much publicity and it was at this point in about December 1941 that a change in procedure occurred. And here we come to another of the myths with which this period is littered. It was commonly believed that as the protests grew they came to the ears of the Führer who ordered an end to the killings. However, be that as it may, the killings did not stop. They simply took on a different form. Many of the writers and articles dealing with this period state that the programme ended. What actually happened was that the same aims were procured by different means. The gas chambers were no longer used and the crematoria also fell into disuse. These were replaced by lethal injections and even starvation, the bodies being disposed of by mass burial.

As far as the psychiatrists were concerned it was business as usual, and the euthanasia programme continued throughout the war. And in Bavaria it continued even until a few days after the war when children were still being murdered. If Hitler did order an end to the euthanasia murders, their continuance only goes to show how determined the psychiatrists were to pursue their own aims regardless of his wishes.

Special Action 14f13

After the State had been relieved of the ghastly burden of so many of these undesirables, mental patients and useless-eaters, the operation, still under the direction of eminent mental health psychiatrists in T4, was expanded under the code of 14f13. From being limited to mental hospitals and institutions it now embraced German and Austrian inmates and Jews in concentration camps who were sick or invalid, usually as a result of the conditions extant in these places. The starting date for the operation of 14f13 appears to have been some time in December 1941. Special commissions composed of psychiatrists attached to the Berlin staff of T4 were dispatched to the concentration camps to clear the medical bays and sick quarters by way of selection of ill and undesirables. Patients selected were usually despatched to one of the six killing centers and disposed of there.

At Auschwitz around this time about 800 patients in the infectious block were sent to death chambers. Testimony was given at Nuremberg after the war by the S.S. camp doctor at Dachau that at the end of 1941 a commission composed of 4 psychiatrists under the leadership of Professor Dr. Werner Heyde, SS Standartenführer and lecturer in neurology and psychiatry at Würzburg University, arrived at the camp and immediately proceeded to their business. They selected several hundred patients incapable of work who were thenceforth transported to the gas chambers and disposed of. The decision for selection rested upon the incapacity of the prisoners to perform work. Jews were disposed of much more easily by the declaration that they were enemies of National Socialism.

Evidence is shown in a letter written by Dr. Fritz Mennecke, a member of this commission dated November 25th, 1941, which he wrote from Buchenwald, another concentration camp which they visited. The letter was addressed to his wife and gave a brief account of his clinical duties on the commission during the day:

At noon we took time off for lunch then we continued our examinations until 4.00 p.m. I examined 105 patients whilst Muller took 78 so that we finished off the first lot of 183 questionnaires. The second lot consisted of 1200 Jews who were not examined and it was enough to pick out from their documents the reason for their arrest and enter it in the questionnaires.

Apart from the people already covered, the action was extended to include adults and children in many Polish asylums. However there is little evidence available to me at this time regarding these particular murders, and this is a very fruitful area to be examined in the future. Apart from the psychiatrists themselves involved in the programme, others also took advantage of the rare opportunity of so many specimens offered them. One of these was a brain specialist Dr. Julius Hailervorden, Director of the Kaiser Wilhelm Institute in Dillenberg, Hessen-Nassau, who had the good luck to be able to obtain hundreds of brains from the killing centers for use in his laboratory. These brains were from mental patients in various institutions who had been killed by carbon monoxide gas. He freely admitted that he himself had initiated this collaboration in the euthanasia programme and stated:

> I heard that they were going to do that, and so I went up to them and told them, 'Look here now, boys (Menschenskinder), if .you are going to kill all these people, at least take the brains out so that the material could be utilised.' They asked me: 'How many can you examine?' and so I told them 'An unlimited number-the more the better.' I gave them the fixatives, jars and boxes, and instructions for removing and fixing the brains, and then they came bringing them in like the delivery van from the furniture company. The Charitable Transport Company for the Sick brought the brains in batches of 150-250 at a time... There was wonderful material among those brains beautiful mental defectives, mal-formations and early infantile diseases. I accepted those brains of course. Where they came from and how they came to me was realty none of my business.

The development of occurrences up to this time shows plainly that there were no limits to the enthusiasm that the psychiatrists in Berlin felt for T4. How patriotic they must have considered themselves when they then decided to put their brave teams into action in the East, to help the wounded in ice and snow. As Dr. Fritz Mennecke told his wife in a letter on 12th January 1942.

> Since the day before yesterday a large delegation from our organisation, headed by Herr Brack, is on the battlefields of the East to help in saving our wounded in the ice and snow. They include doctors, clerks, nurses, and male nurses from Hadamar and Sonnenstein, a whole detachment of 20-30 persons. **This is a top secret.** Only those persons who could not be spared were excluded. Professor Nitsche regrets that the staff of our institution at Eichberg had to be taken away so soon.[9]

This quote speaks for itself, when one considers who was "helping" the wounded in ice and snow. It becomes evident that the German soldiers in the East had to fight three fronts: the Russian Army, the partisans and the enemies in their own ranks. As if the war-killing had not been enough, now special committees were put into action to relieve the wounded German soldiers from their painful existence. The soldiers thus were not only in a fix strategically, but also morally as well; if they were wounded, how would they be "helped"?

---

[9] Editor: the emphasized text was in Schreiber's original.

CHAPTER VII

THE PSYCHIATRIC FINAL SOLUTION TO THE JEWISH QUESTION

The Nazi extermination camps need to be clearly distinguished from the concentration camps opened a few months after the Nazi accession to power with the establishment of Dachau (near Munich). The extermination camps had not followed in the line of progression of the concentration camps, but had a quite separate evolution of their own, which up to now has puzzled many students of the subject. However, with what we know about psychiatric plans we can fit the apparently unprecedented in its place in the logical sequence of the psychiatric-eugenic programme. The extermination camps, the apex of development on the sterilization, castration, and euthanasia chain of evolution could be considered to be the full flowering of the plans laid by the psychiatrists and on the basis of experience gained in the euthanasia programme were the perfection of murder on assembly line basis.

The names of the camps were Belsec, Treblinka, Sobibor and Chelmno and they were established between 1941 and 1943. A number of features distinguish these extermination camps from the better known concentration camps including the following:

1. They were all situated in Poland usually in a desolate, virtually uninhabited area.
2. Their only purpose was to kill Jews as quickly, efficiency, economically, and profitably as possible.
3. Although being run on the spot by the SS and their auxiliaries, daily orders came from a different source.

Without going into too many horrifying details, it would be as well to give a brief picture of how the extermination camps operated.

The camps resembled very closely a mass-production line in a modern industrial plant. Nothing was wasted. When a transport full of Jewish victims rolled into the nearby station the "passengers" were herded into the camp and had to surrender their valuables and currency supposedly for safe-keeping. They were then taken to changing rooms where they stripped, their clothes being later sent to a charity relief in Germany, and were horse-whipped into the death chambers and gassed. When they were all dead the doors were opened and bodies pulled out and hosed down by the Jewish commandos, mouths were inspected, gold teeth removed and later remitted to the Reichsbank and the various cavities of the body were explored for other hidden valuables.

Prior to the gassing, of course, the hair had been shaved from the heads of the women. This had been found to be very useful for knitting felt slippers for U-boat crews. Having searched the corpses for valuables they were then loaded into railway wagons and taken to the crematorium. After burning, the bones were ground in a bone-crushing mill and sacked up, ashes also being put in sacks and both of these sent back to Germany to be used as fertiliser. There was even a formula for their use: 1 layer of ashes 1 layer of bone and 1 layer of earth.

Although there are a number of other cases on record, I shall give just two examples which show where the orders for the camps came from. On August 7-8, 1946, at Nuremberg, Sturmbannführer Georg Konrad Morgen, an SS judge gave evidence on behalf of the SS as an indicted organisation. Morgen had been transferred in July 1943 from the SS Military Courts to the Criminal Police at Himmler's request. His job was the investigation of embezzlement in concentration camps. In following up cases of corruption in the camps, he stumbled upon some top secret evidence.

Morgen's argument at the Nuremberg trials was that the extermination camps were not run by the SS at all. Apparently in the summer of 1943 he heard from the commander of the Security Police and SD in the Lublin region of Poland that there had been a wedding in a Jewish labour camp which had been attended by 1100 guests including many German SS men. Morgen, amazed at this weird tale, looked further and in doing so came across another camp, "rather peculiar and impenetrable" which was run by Christian Wirth, who confirmed the story of the Jewish wedding and explained that it was part of a plan by which Wirth hoped to persuade Jews to serve in the camps where they would assist in the exterminations.

Although the four camps had been mentioned earlier in the Nuremberg trials, this was the first clue concerning their ultimate headquarters. Morgen insisted that the administration of the camps was actually not in SS hands, having seen Wirth's daily orders. These did not come from Himmler's Office but from the Führer's Chancellery (T4) and had been signed "Blankenberg." Morgen's evidence was the only clue to the true command lines of the Jewish extermination programme.

This was confirmed years later in the recent trial of the notorious Franz Stangl. He was an Austrian policeman who automatically became a member of the Austrian Gestapo following the Anschluss. In November 1940 he was transferred to the General Foundation for institutional Care, one of the T4 front groups. He was told to report to a Dr. Werner at the Reichskriminalpolizeiamt in Berlin.

Werner told him that he'd been selected for a very difficult and demanding job of police superintendent at a special institute administered by the Foundation. Werner explained to him that both Russia and America had for some time had a law which allowed them to carry out mercy killings (this of course was not true) on people who were insane or badly deformed. He explained that a law was going to be passed in Germany in the near future but it was going to be done only after a great deal of psychological preparation. However, in the meantime the task had begun under absolute secrecy.

He then went on to explain that the patients selected for the action were carefully examined and a series of tests were carried out by at least two physicians and only those absolutely incurable were put to a totally painless death. Stangl was told that all he had to do was to be responsible for law and order in the institute and not actually involved in the operation himself, this being carried out entirely by doctors. He was to be responsible for maintaining maximum security.

After his talk with Werner, Stangl reported to the KdF. He recalled that he thought it was Brack who greeted him at T4, explained to him his specific police duties and left him the choice of where he should be posted. He decided to be posted to Austria where he would be near his family. He was given a telephone number and the name of a village where he was to go and make a 'phone call and would be given instructions.' He carried out the instructions for making contact and was driven to Hartheim.

After arrival he met the doctors and Captain Christian Wirth, who was his superior in his duties. Wirth apparently didn't bother too much with the scientific justifications that the psychiatrists employed, because as he said, sentimental slobber about such people made him puke. The two chief medical officers were Dr. Lohnauer and Dr. Renno and in addition to these there were 14 nurses; 7 men and 7 women. Hartheim was set up and run as a hospital where examinations were given and Stangl's job was to see that such things as identity papers and certificates for the mental patients were dealt with and done correctly.

After Hartheim, Stangl took a brief tour of duty at another euthanasia institute, Bernberg and after that was told to report back to T4 to get new orders. in the interview he was informed that he had a choice either to return to his former police post (where he hadn't in fact got on very welt with his superiors) or go to Lublin, in Poland. He decided on the latter and was told to report to Higher SS and Police Chief Odilo Globocnik at SS Headquarters, Lublin. Globocnik gave him the task of building a new extermination camp — Sobibor.

Shortly after his arrival at the site that was to be Sobibor, personnel from the "euthanasia action" started to arrive. Amongst them were many old friends from Hartheim and work started on the camp which Stangl was to command from May until August 1942, when he took over Treblinka until August 1943.

Although he was able to evade justice after the war he was finally caught and sentenced in 1970 to life imprisonment for co-responsibility in the murder of 400,000 men, women and children in Treblinka during the year of his command. It is difficult to arrive at even approximate totals of the number of men, women and children who died in these camps but the following figures from the Polish Commission for War Crimes will give some idea of the enormity of the crime:

Treblinka	....	700,000-800,000
Sobibor	....	over 250,000
Belzec	....	almost 600,000
Chelmno	....	over 300,000

Interestingly some of the "students" trained in the murder schools were later traced to the extermination camps, 130 to Belzec, 106 to Sobibor and 90 to Treblinka. Many of these had learned their skills in Hartheim.

As the tide of war turned in the East there was much activity to prevent the camps falling into Russian hands and being exploited by them for propaganda purposes. Elaborate precautions were taken to avoid this by razing the sites level and generally altering the landscape by planting trees and shrubs, etc. Personnel of the camps were dispersed to high risk war areas. Wirth himself is believed to have been killed by partisans in Yugoslavia in 1944.

Amongst the "bureaucrats of death" there was the inevitable scramble to evade the Allied armies as they closed in on the Reich. Some were successful, others not. Philip Bouhler committed suicide as the Russians approached Berlin and Leonardo Conti also in his cell at Nuremberg. Karl Brandt was caught, sentenced and executed.

The Limburg trial planned in 1961 was concerned with some of the top psychiatrists and bureaucrats, one of whom was the eminent psychiatrist Professor Dr. Werner Heyde, super expert in T4. In the preceding years he had adopted an alias, being known as Dr. Sawade and had practised openly in Germany. He had done a variety of work for a state insurance agency, and law courts. Many people, including judges, prosecutors, physicians, university professors and high state officials knew his identity. And they preserved the conspiracy of silence. Whilst awaiting trial he attempted to escape. Five days before the trial at a time when he was left unguarded, he committed suicide.

His co-defendants in the trial also managed to escape justice. Dr. Friedrich Tillman, for 10 years prior to 1945 [the] Director of Cologne orphanages, jumped (or was pushed) from a tenth-storey window; another Dr. Bohne escaped on the Nazi escape-route to South America. The fourth Defendant, Dr. Hans Hefelmann, chief of section IIb ("mercy killing") in the Chancellery of the Führer was declared medically unable to stand trial due to illness. it seems that people in high places didn't want these trials to take place.

Another personality who was questioned during the preparation of the same trial was Dr. Werner Villinger, who has been credited with being instrumental in starting the mental hygiene movement in pre-war Germany, and re-starting the same movement as a mental health movement after the war. An eminent psychiatrist who, two years before Hitler came to power, had advocated the sterilization of patients with hereditary diseases, he was convinced that the roots of what we call temperament and character lay deep in the inherited constitution. At the time of his questioning for the Limburg trial it became known publicly that he was implicated in the euthanasia murders in a prominent and very active role. He went into the mountains and committed suicide. A former colleague and assistant of his Dr. Helmut Ehrhardt, in an obituary published in the journal "Der Nervenarzt" [The Nerve Doctor] explained Dr. Villager's sad demise as an accident and with much sorrow, regretted his passing, and mourned the loss for humanity of such a wonderful and humane man.

However, for those who survived the war, did not commit suicide, and were still at large, there was at least one place where they could appear with impunity in an understanding community who welcomed their talents and shared their viewpoint.

CHAPTER VIII

THE PHOENIX

Especially since the last world war we have done much to infiltrate the various social organisations throughout the country, and in their work and in their point of view one can see clearly how the principles for which this society and others stood in the past have become accepted as part of the ordinary working plan of these various bodies. That is as it should be, and while we can take heart from this we must be healthily discontented and realize that there is still more work to be done along this line. Similarly we have made a useful attack upon a number of professions. The two easiest of them naturally are the teaching profession and the Church: the two most difficult are law and medicine...

If we are to infiltrate the professional and social activities of other people I think we must imitate the Totalitarians and organize some kind of fifth column activity!

John Rawlings Rees M.D.

Address to the Annual Meeting of the National Council for Mental Hygiene, June 18th, 1940.

During the war the name of Eugenics became even more heavily associated with the Nazis and consequently afterwards a whitewashing procedure began, the first step of which was the reconstitution of the various National Councils of Mental Hygiene. The first to be re-founded was the British National Association for Mental Health. But before we go into detail on this a bit of history is important.

Montagu Norman had been Governor of the Bank of England for many years. He and his right hand man, Otto Niemeyer (of German origin), had persistently backed the re-arming of Germany [and] made loans to Germany and encouraged the financiers of the City of London to do the same. Norman supported and financed Germany's cause right up until the Declaration of War.

When German troops crashed into Czechoslovakia in September 1938, Germany claimed Czech assets. They applied through the Bank for International Settlements, of which Norman was a Director, for the release of Czech gold held in the Bank of England.

The financial tomfoolery that followed would leave anyone confused, but the outcome was that £6,000,000 worth of Czech gold was transferred to Hitler's Government, released by Norman.

Before the war, Norman attended the christening of the son of his comrade-in-arms, Dr. Hjalmar Schacht, Minister of Finance and President of the Reichsbank, and in July 1942 was suspected of having visited Schacht in Germany during the War. This alleged visit has always been dismissed by stating that Schacht was in fact being held in a concentration camp for disagreeing with Hitler, and obviously Norman would have been unable to visit him there. The documents of the Nuremberg Trials, however, show quite clearly that Schacht had only been sent to the concentration camp in 1944 — more than two years after the suspected visit by Norman. Whether or not he visited Schacht remains a mystery but that he did financially support Germany is a recorded fact.

Norman had married Priscilla Koch de Gooreynd (now Lady Norman) who was a disciple of Dame Evelyn Fox, a long-standing member of the eugenics society. In her own words, she was completely dedicated to Evelyn Fox. And so Priscilla Norman had been working in the Mental Hygiene movement since the 20's.

Recommendations had been put forward by Lord Feversham in the week that War broke out, that the Central Association for Mental Welfare; The National Council for Mental Hygiene and the Mental After Care-Association should amalgamate into one Association. So, for the duration of the war a Provisional Association for Mental Health was formed under the Chairmanship of Lady Norman.

At the end of the war Montagu and Priscilla Norman gave themselves whole-heartedly to the establishment of such an Association. as Lord Feversham had suggested, in which the related organisations were amalgamated. As Montagu had retired in 1944, he dedicated himself completely to his wife's scheme and complemented her methods with his own. From meetings at Thorpe Lodge, the home of the Normans, the National Association for

Mental Health became a reality and the framework for similar changes to take place in the rest of the world. Otto Niemeyer was made Treasurer, and the next phase began.

Upon the invitation of the NAMH, the international Committee for Mental Hygiene held a congress at the Ministry of Health in London, where it formally established itself under the new name, World Federation for Mental Health — WFMH. It became the international coordinator for national Mental Health and Mental Hygiene groups in many countries of the world, and besides a new name, the meeting initiated a change in the direction of its activities.

Already we see the strong involvement of the NAMH in the WFMH, and in future history the NAMH succeeded in exerting considerable influence in the activities of the WFMH.

Lady Norman was appointed to the Executive Board of WFMH and with Otto Niemeyer's niece, Mary Appleby, as the General Secretary of the British NAMH, the chain was complete. Miss Appleby s previous experience in the German Section of the British Foreign Office would serve her well.

The first elected president of the WFMH was Dr. John Rawlings Rees, a British psychiatrist who was quoted at the beginning of this chapter. The full lecture details a plan whereby each mental hygienist operates as a lone-agent, constantly feeding propaganda to private individuals and groups without naming the Mental Hygiene movement as the true sponsor.

He asks that constant propaganda be fed to and pressure put on: Universities, Educational Establishments, Medicine, Press, Parliament, Magazines and Weeklies, Literary figures, Film makers, medical students, civil servants and trades union leaders. To obtain the goals of the Mental Hygiene movement, without the movement ever being named.

In 1948, when he was elected Chairman of the WFMH he accepted the position on this newly-formed august body. The congress at which the WFMH was inaugurated was the Third International Congress on Mental Health. A Vice-President of the Congress was Dr. Carl G. Jung who had been described by Dr. Conti as "representing German psychiatry under the Nazis." He had been co-editor of the Journal for Psychotherapy with Dr. M.H. Goering, the cousin of Marshal Hermann Goering. There is definite evidence that Dr. Goering was fully cognizant of the euthanasia murders. Another of the German delegates to the 1948 congress was Dr.

Friedrich Mauz, Professor of Psychiatry at Koenigsburg University. He denied his connection to the euthanasia programme, without condemning it, by indicating that his invitation to a euthanasia conference was no conclusive evidence of his complicity in any such activities.

Dr Adolf Wahlmann, a noted psychiatrist in the European League for Mental Hygiene would have attended if he had not previously stood trial and been imprisoned for the murder of Polish and other labourers in his institution, Hadamar, which had already been emptied by the mass-murder of all the patients contained therein. As already mentioned, Hadamar Institution trained many of the extermination camp officers on special assignments by T4. Among them there was a man called Gomerski who was engaged in mass killings at Treblinka and Sobibor with such skill, as a result of his training, that he was nicknamed "The Doctor".

Thanks to the propaganda and social education of the eugenicists and mental healers, the killing of mental patients has never been considered a terribly serious matter, and Wahlmann, a mass-murderer, was released in 1954.

Dr. Paul Nitsche would also have attended, as he was a leading member of the Mental Hygiene movement, had it not been for the fact that he was executed for the mass-murder of mental patients in 1947.

Shortly, other surviving members of the old gang began to gather in the WFMH.

Dr Werner Villinger had, after the war become a world-famous psychiatrist. His specialities included juvenile delinquency, child guidance and group therapy. He was also Professor of Psychiatry at Marburg and a very important member of the WFMH. He sat on the US White House Conference on Children and Youth. In the conference of the WFMH on Health and Human Relations which took place in Hiddesen-near-Detmold in 1951, he was co-chairman together with Rees. In 1952 he was a member of a WFMH group on Educating the Public which met during the Annual Conference in Brussels. Doris Odlum, late member of the Eugenics Society and Miss Appleby, already mentioned were Chairman and Secretary respectively of the group.

In 1961, German Federal Authorities caught up with Villinger and after three preliminary sessions prior to the Limburg trial, as we have seen already, he threw himself off a mountain top near Innsbruck to his death. His apologist and author of his obituary, Dr. Ehrhardt, was also an active member of the WFMH.

In the book *Contemporary European Psychiatry* (a book on different psychiatric practices in Europe) which was published in 1961 in the United States and Europe, the Austrian psychiatrist Dr. Hans Hoff claims in his chapter on Germany and Austria, that sterilization of mentally ill was a scientific procedure so long as a psychiatrist was adviser to the Eugenic Courts.

[Like] Ehrhard, Hoff praises the work of Villinger. Hoff was an active supporter of the WFMH, and in 1959 he became its President. Shortly after Ehrhardt's whitewash of Villinger's suicide, Hoff attempted an even trickier whitewash job, in a preface to Ehrhardt's book "Euthanasie und Vernichtung Lebensunwerten Lebens" (Euthanasia and the Destruction of 'Life-unworthy' Life) and he gives it full approval. Basically, they confused the whole issue by pointing out that the question of euthanasia is still a medical and moral one. In 1968, Ehrhardt was elected to the Executive Board of the WFMH. The book was favorably reviewed in an American psychiatric journal.

Ehrhardt also praised Dr. Max de Crinis as a "courageous and energetic physician" and spoke of the "comparatively few mental patients" killed. De Crinis had of course been one the T4 advisers. His former assistant, Dr. Muller-Hegemann, was left behind the Iron Curtain after the Second World War ended. However, even so daunting a situation could not halt the course of progress and by 1969 Dr. Muller-Hegemann had been elected to the Executive Board of the WFMH.

The supporters of the eugenic movement from all over the world who had backed the mass-murders morally, streamed into the WFMH and its member associations at an alarming rate, and yesterday's euthanasiasts became today's Mental Healthists. Some of them kept their membership card of the Eugenics Society others let it drop, but didn't forget its ideals. Others again, to be fair, must have realized their error and disappeared from the picture, but this was only a small percentage.

In Great Britain the eugenically oriented salvationists who became active mental health supporters were:

Dr. Doris Odlum; Dr. E. Slater; Sir Aubrey Lewis; Dr. Lancelot Hogben; Miss Robina Addis; Lord and Lady Adrian; Lord Brain; Sir Russell Brain; Prof. C. Fraser Brockington; Dr. Felix W. Brown; Rt. Hon. Sir John Brunner; Prof. Cyril Burt; Comdr. and Mrs. B.R. Darwin; Lady Darwin; Prof. H.J. Eysenck; The Earl of Feversham; Miss Evelyn Fox; Dame Katherine Furse; The Earl of Iveagh; Dr. F.M. Martin; Dr. T.A. Munro; Lady Petrie; Dr. R.E. Pilkington; Kenneth Robinson; The Rt. Hon. Lord Justice Scott; Mrs H.M. Strickland; Prof. J.M. Tanner; Prof. Sir G.H. Thomson; Prof. R.M. Titmuss; Dr. J. Tizard; Dr. A.F. Tredgold; Dr. R.F. Tredgold; Dr. Isabel G.H. Wilson; Prof. R.C. Wofinden; Dr. T.L. Pilkington.

In West Germany:
Dr. Werner Villinger (T4-adviser); Dr. Carl Jung; Dr. Werner Heyde (T4-adviser); Dr. Ehrhard (Villinger's Assistant).

In East Germany:
Dr. Muller-Hegemann (De Crinis Assistant).

The German Society for Mental Hygiene, however, was dissolved, its members scattered for cover and its reports left incomplete. Until today no new German Society has been founded on a national basis.

Villinger had tried to collect the Mental Hygiene movement back into one group, but the murderers were not willing to come together in a German society, where they could easily be isolated as a cancer. Instead they preferred the mask of a group from which they could direct similar campaigns on each country in the world, just as they had done before. Their names are still to be found amongst the professors for psychiatry at the universities, the staff in scientific research institutes, and among the members of professional associations.

In Austria:
Professor Hans Hoff.

In Canada:
Dr. Karl Stern (who studied in Germany under Ernst Rüdin).

In Denmark:

Dr. Georg K. Stürup; Dr Pout Bonnevie; Dr. Paul J. Reiter; Dr. Erik Strömgren; Dr. Einar Geert-Jorgensen; Dr August Wimmer; Dr Kurt Fremming; Dr. Jens Chr. Smidt; Dr. Tage Kemp; Dr. Max Schmidt; Dr. G.E. Schroder.

In Norway:

Dr. Jan Mohr; Dr. J. Schutz-Larsen.

In the USA:

Dr. Walter C. Alvarez.

In each of these countries, and in others, a National Association for Mental Health or an equivalent group existed which was recruited into the fold by the WFMH.

In Denmark, Louis Grandjean who had been Director of the Landsforeningen for Mentalhygiejne for 5 1/2 years wrote in 1954 "The Little Milieu" which was a study in family heredity. In the book he praises Herman Lundborg and Sören Hansen both notorious vice-presidents of the international Federation of Eugenic Organisations.

Stürup, of the Danish "Landsforeningen," also had an interesting career. Immediately after the war he undertook a psychiatric study of Danes who had collaborated with the Nazis. The records and results on Stürup's insistence were declared secret. The effect is that these results are not available to the public and no-one can identify the Nazi collaborators and what happened to them.

In 1960, Eggert Petersen, former psychological-warfare operative in Danish Military Intelligence, was appointed director of the Danish "Landsforeningen." This may not be significant but it bears an amazing resemblance to the British NAMH.

The professional associations of medical men and psychiatrists were not immediately recruited, as the Board of the WFMH over the years contained many of the top men from these same professional associations. Influence was easily brought to bear on the American Psychiatric Association, the Association of Neurologists and Psychiatrists, the Deutsche Gesellschaft für Psychiatrie und Nervenheilkunde (Marburg), the Australian and New Zealand College of Psychiatrists, the Canadian Psychiatric Association and many more. Today many of these associations have joined the

WFMH ranks of member and affiliated associations. There remain only a few professional groups in the mental sciences who are not swayed by the hypnotic command to "Kill".

The influence of a huge professional body could not be halted by the mere death of over a quarter of a million mental patients and others, and at least a million Jews in the T4 extermination camps, it could only be slowed; but the ranks are reforming for the next social onslaught which this time may not be disguised by war but by charity. Lord Adrian, member of the Eugenics Society, the British NAMH and the Voluntary Euthanasia Society, expressed this kind of charity in a speech he gave in 1956:

> ...preventive health services are bound to interfere with individual liberty... and if they aim at mental as well as physical health they must be prepared to separate mothers from children and to supervise the lives of people who would like to be let alone.

CHAPTER IX

THE SAME OLD TUNE

In the meantime the Eugenics Society in England had gone underground. The 1945 Annual Report shows that the Society would no longer undertake direct propaganda to public or Parliament, but only to related organisations. From this moment on the Eugenics Society became a hidden element, delineating the propaganda lines of other organisations.

In 1957, Dr. C.P. Blacker, then Honorary Secretary of the Society, suggested a further retreat into the background, and adherence to the policy of crypto-Eugenics, that is, through finance and propaganda from behind the scenes.

This proposal was adopted in 1960 and the Society set out on a wide-spread programme of manipulation. Genetics and Eugenics as such — not behind the cloak of mental health — were still, in spite of their unsavory associations in the public mind, able to make remarkable progress. And the various eugenics societies flourish today.

Some of the well-known arms of the octopus are: The Marie Stopes Memorial Foundation, a subsidiary subsidized bit the Eugenics Society; the Family Planning Association and the International Planned Parenthood Foundation, which are heavily financed by the Eugenics Society; the Voluntary Sterilization Association was directed from the same address as the Eugenics Society; the Galton Foundation, run by the Eugenics Society; and others.

Dr. C.P. Blacker, now chairman of the Eugenics Society discovered, while a member of a committee of investigation on the atrocities committed by Nazi doctors, that although none of the experiments produced scientific conclusions and although the methods used by the Nazis were unfortunate, euthanasia of the insane was acceptable.

In an address to the Eugenics Society in 1951 he outlined the three following areas in relation to Germany:

1. Sterilization under the 1934 edict of law.
2. Euthanasia of the chronically mentally ill and of those similarly handicapped.
3. Experiments using live people for the purpose of developing an economical method of mass sterilization.

He acknowledged that he was quite satisfied with the area of legal sterilization, the law governing which he thought was correct, except for sterilization based on racial grounds — for Blacker naturally makes no attempt to pass moral judgment.

On the subject of euthanasia of the mentally ill he explains:

> ...these people were mercifully killed. The idea of merciful killing is not unknown in this country; in fact a society on a voluntary basis... exists to promote it.

Nevertheless, he condemns experiments on living people for three specific reasons:

a) It was not necessary to use human beings. Animal experiments would have met the purpose just as well.
b) No results of the slightest scientific interest are recorded; nor in my opinion were any likely to have resulted even if more time had been available.
c) The experiments failed in their primary purpose of providing a cheap method of mass sterilization or castration...

If we examine this condemnation more closely, it is easily recognized that had it been the case that an economical means of mass sterilization had been discovered, the experiments could only have been condemned by reason of the first-named point. Apart from that, these three viewpoints implied that the development of a low-cost method of mass sterilization would represent a worthwhile scientific product. Where and under what conditions could such a wonderful achievement be put to use? As if wishing to pursue his unspoken, logical train of thought, he recommends that the continuation of experimentation with one of the sterilization-drugs which were being used by the Nazi doctors would be perfectly in order.

The profound and immeasurable silence of the medical profession in regard to the German doctors does not find its foundation on a lack of knowledge about what happened.

Today, sterilizations as well as euthanasia are encouraged for eugenic reasons by medical people, mainly psychiatrists, but of course now dressed in different garb. Just as the master builders of T4 went underground after the war and later emerged as members of the WFMH, so also did their ideals and their interests.

Eugenics has made a comeback as a so-called experimental field whose products are test-tube babies, artificial insemination, and the like. Articles in the popular press, about artificial insemination and genetic engineering in the future, are very common today. Sterilization has been resuscitated as part of the Planned Parenthood Programme. Whereas formerly one heard the cry, "If we don't do something soon we'll be inundated by people", and Malthus proclaimed, "If we don t control birth we'll run out of supplies of food", nowadays the call goes out, "If we don't start using birth control, we won t have anywhere to stand." The melody is the same, only the words have changed.

Euthanasia has surfaced again as a charitable organisation dispensing "Death with Dignity", a new euphemism, with the aim of giving a person who is in a state of health which precludes any chance of being cured the opportunity of letting himself be killed, but of course only when he is complete agreement with the measure. In the case of mental unbalance, a relative can give consent. Once again the first signs of forced euthanasia are becoming visible, aimed at the mentally ill.

Should anyone be interested in getting a picture of the current situation, he should have a look around his home country, and at neighbouring ones, for he will surely find something along the lines of:

1. A (national) association for Mental Health
2. A Eugenics society or group
3. Some type of Abortion Reform League
4. An association for Voluntary Sterilization
5. An association for Voluntary Euthanasia

If the members and committees of these associations are then cross-checked, he will see that:

1. Many names cross-check
2. A large percentage of the members of branches 3, 4, and 5 above stem from sections 1 and 2.
3. They constantly carry on mutual complementary propaganda.

Take Great Britain as a concrete example. The directorate of the Abortion Law Reform Association is comprised of:

Prof. Glanville Williams NAMH supporter and member of the Eugenics Society.
Sir Julian Huxley NAMH supporter, an officer of the Eugenics Society and of the Euthanasia Society.
Baroness Stocks member of the NAMH Galton Lecturer.
Dr Eliot Slater member of the Eugenics Society — and many others.

The Executive Committee of the Euthanasia Society:

Lord Adrian member of the NAMH and of the Eugenics Society.
Prof. Glanville Williams member of the NAMH and of the Eugenics Society.
Sir Julian Huxley member of the NAMH and of the Eugenics Society.

On the executive committee of the Birth Control Campaign figure among others:

Prof. Eliot Slater member of the Eugenics Society.
Baroness Stocks member of the NAMH and of the Eugenics Society.
Prof. Glanville Williams member of the Eugenics Society and of the NAMH.

Why this should be, the author doesn't know, but it is the medical men of such groups who provide the "scientific" rationale and methodology to justify and achieve the desired ends. In the U.S.A. in 1968 a voluntary euthanasia bill was introduced in Florida and an eminent surgeon and member of the American Medical Association — AMA — argued the case for it:

A bill to be entitled

An act relating to the right to die with dignity; providing an effective date.

Be It Enacted by the Legislature of the State of Florida:

Section 1. All natural persons are equal before the law and have inalienable rights, among them the right to enjoy and defend life and liberty, to be permitted to die with dignity, to pursue happiness, to be rewarded for industry, and to acquire possess and protect property. No person shall be deprived of any right because of race religion or national origin.

Section 2. Any person with the same formalities as required by law for the execution of a last will and testament, may execute a document directing that he shall have the right to death with dignity, and that his life shall not be prolonged beyond the point of a meaningful existence.

Section 3. in the event any person is unable to make such a decision because of mental or physical incapacity, a spouse or person or persons of first degree kinship shall be allowed to make such a decision, provided written consent is obtained from:

1. The spouse or person of first degree kinship or
2. in the event of two (2) persons of first degree kinship both such persons or
3. in the event of three (3) or more persons of first degree kinship the majority of those persons.

Section 4. If any person is disabled and there is no kinship as provided in section 3, death with dignity shall be granted any person if in the opinion of three (3) physicians the prolongation of life is meaningless.

Section 5. Any document executed hereunder must be recorded with the clerk of the circuit court in order to be effective.

Section 6. This act shall take effect upon becoming law.

Fortunately this bill was not passed, and so far the AMA has been silent on the whole issue, but judging by the silence with which the German atrocities were met I can safety predict that the AMA will soon be unofficially espousing the cause of voluntary euthanasia.

In 1935, the editor of the Journal of the American Medical Association observed that the average doctor frequently faced the problem (of euthanasia) when it was a matter between him and his patient and he could decide in his own way without any interference.

The principles and practices are exactly the same as those that the Nazi psychiatrists used. One British expert recently arguing the case for euthanasia even went so tar as to say that certain defectives are a burden to themselves and others (the State perhaps) and therefore should be put out of their misery.

South Africa

With the full support of the South African Council for Mental Health and the Association of Neurologists and Psychiatrists, South Africa, which is heavily inclined in this direction anyway, will have sterilization laws introduced before long. At this time heavy propaganda for sterilization is being promoted there as a continuation of S. Africa's early history. In 1930, H.B. Fantham, Professor of Zoology at Witwatersrand, wrote in Child Welfare Magazine:

> "...there must be limitations of multiplication of those definitely inferior or below average in inborn good qualities. In South Africa there must be limitations of the 'poor white' element."

In 1934 Dr. P.W. Laidler, Medical Officer for Health of East London, wrote an article for the "S.A. Tydskrif vir Geneeskundiges" called for a South African sterilization law "on the lines of Germany." Some interesting quotes from his article:

> "It is the white man's deficients who drag him down."

> "The prevention of family is essential where stock is poor."

> "A lessening of the increase of the unfit would lighten the tax payer's burden."

"We are overburdened with poor of normal minds and defectives. Possibly we are overburdened with better class minds."

"Man continues to load himself with a burden of deficients."

In October 1971, as this book was being written, Dr. Troskie an Executive member of the South African Medical and Dental Council, called for the merciless elimination of weak genetic elements. He proposed the formation of a Genetic Committee composed of a judge and medical, sociological and religious experts to:

"prevent those parents from leaving a burden on society. The committee will make the decision for them."

This is apparently not a new idea in South Africa, as several groups are involved in a debate over whether there should be compulsory or voluntary sterilization, and now a group of sociologists intend to approach the Prime Minister about the problem.

The parallel between Nazi Germany and modern South Africa is very close.

U.S.A.

The Rockefeller institute that backs the AMA has produced devastating results at home and overseas. It was Rockefeller who financed the foundation of the Kaiser Wilhelm Institute, and gave Professor Rüdin one whole floor of the building for his genetic research in the 20's. The German Mental Hygiene Movement was heavily subsidized by Rockefeller and thereby put into a healthy position to continue its aims and objectives to the bitter end. Further it was Dr. Alexis Carrel of the Rockefeller institute and a Nobel Prize Winner who so loudly applauded the actions of the Germans and blatantly advocated the mass murder of mental patients and prisoners.

Currently in the U.S. the psychiatric profession is making extensive use of prisoners as experimental material for medical experiments with AMA approval. The Rockefeller family continues to subsidize the Medical-Psychiatric professors and one of the Rockefellers is on the Board of the American National Association for Mental Health. In 1970 in Hawaii, a bill was introduced the exact wording of which was:

A Bill for an Act Relating to Population Control.

Section 1:

The legislation finds

1. that population growth is the most serious and most challenging problem for mankind today;
2. that the time necessary for the population of the world to double is now about thirty-five years;
3. that the "death rate solution" by war famine or pestilence is an unacceptable destructive solution to the problem of birth control;
4. that population control is an acceptable humanitarian solution to the problem of population growth. The purpose of this Act is to control the population size of this State by a program of birth regulation.

Section 2:
Every physician attending a woman resident of this State at the time she is giving birth in the State shall, it the woman has two or more living children, perform such medical technique or operation as will render the woman sterile.

Section 3:

This Act shall take effect on July 1, 1971.

Even amongst our neighbors trends in this direction can be recognized. In Switzerland,it was Dr. André Repond who had applauded Germany's efforts, and had been so proud of his own work in ensuring that only eugenically sound marriages took place in one of the Swiss cantons.

The question of euthanasia and sterilization are not problems of yesterday to be discussed at club-meetings or amongst intellectuals as philosophic or historic subjects. The psychiatrists, as strong as ever, have begun to agitate more and more loudly for the right to sterilize and kill.

In July 1972 Dr. T.L. Pilkington in "The Practitioner" called for yet further murders to be committed.

> ...there seem to be clear indications that technologically developed nations will be rapidly obliged to review the complexity of the life that they create, embark on a modern eugenic programme designed to steepen the tail of the graph of the normal I.Q. distribution below 100 or consider some form of legalised euthanasia. It is possible, of course, that the final 'solution' will combine all these with increasing methods of specific prevention.

The Death March has again begun.

Author's Note

When I decided to write this book, I intended simply to record the events in Germany as a warning against similar occurrences which could take place in other countries. Shortly after I had begun to familiarize myself with the subject, I realized that I faced a problem which had already reached international proportions and which had even then deeply entrenched itself in Great Britain. I spent 5 years in England and overseas in order to research the information which I am now making public.

Perhaps I ought to have written two books; perhaps I should have proceeded with my investigations until every volume was fully documented — I do not know.

Yet the fact remains that the psychiatrists and "socially conscious" groups whose hands are stained with the blood of millions of people, and who have created an atmosphere in which similar events could happen in every other part of the world, are still alive today, and are pursuing the same professions as before, only in a form that is more disguised.

This book would not contain as much material about England if my enquiries had not led me there.

Others may feel the desire to carry my work further — and I would honestly like to stimulate this.

The current activities of psychiatrists must be seen in a new light when we take into consideration the fact that their allegedly charitable goals could be a cloak of Invisibility designed to camouflage their ominous purposes in the face of their fellow men.

The psychiatrists began early on to bring their own private secret service to life and to infiltrate governments. I do not wish to elucidate in detail the oft-mentioned theory that Hitler was brought to power through the action of a secret group. For those who want to do further research into this, this book may be of considerable direct importance.

In the "Archives for Racial and Social Biology," Volume 25, 1931, the psychiatrist Prof. F. Lenz clarifies Hitler's *Mein Kampf.* He quotes Hitler abundantly, and establishes that Hitler is the man to finally grant Racial Hygiene its rightful place.

The conveniently accepted opinion is that Hitler was the embodiment of all evil who forced his subjects against their will to perform the historically "singular" atrocities of the Third Reich. This consideration is not only imperfect: it also leads deliberately away from the facts and twists them.

It seems impossible that one man could draw 60 million people under his spell, and make them indifferent to such mass slaughter as was brought about by the psychiatrists under the Third Reich, without some support; even if only from some private interest group.

From the article by Lenz it is obvious how the would-be mass butchers, favored by Hitler at least since 1931, had already carried out moral reconditioning on their stout-hearted puppet. For Lenz himself says in this article about *Mein Kampf,* "Naturally the ideas which Hitler outlines here are not new." No, they certainly were not new, but with Hitler as a puppet, the psychiatrists for the first time found themselves in the position of being able to transform their secret objectives and interests into reality. Lenz closes his article with the words:

> I would like to sum up by saying: Hitler is the first politician of really great influence who has recognized Racial Hygiene as a principal obligation for all politics, and who wants to stand up for it energetically.

Whether or not psychiatry was the sole private interest group which aided Hitler to power has yet to be explored in detail. It is a fact that Hitler took their watchwords literally. However, even the psychiatrists themselves did not have so tight a grip on Hitler as to make him give them a free hand for their mass murders, for they had to go about their murder activities behind his back and without his direct consent.

Hitler had barely come to power when the "Deutsche Verband für psychische Hygiene" (German Union for Mental Health), at a session held on the 16th of July, 1933, changed not only its name to the "Deutscher Verband far psychische Hygiene und Rassenhygiene" (German institute for Mental Health and Racial Hygiene) but also its officers. Prof. Dr. Sommer stepped back and Hitler-supporter Ernst Rüdin took over the leadership.

It is evident from the memorial notice published by Rüdin for the deceased Ploetz in the "Archiv für Rassen und Gesellschaftsbiologie" (Archives for Racial and Social Biology), 1940, Volume I, just how much Hitler had taken up the racial hygiene theories of his masters. Rüdin writes:

> It is tragic fate that Ploetz is no longer alive to witness the solution to the problem of understanding and co-operation among the Nordic peoples, he, who believed so unshakeably in the resolute leadership of Adolf Hitler and in his holy mission of national and international racial hygiene.

Hitler was an evil man and no one would want to assert that he was not responsible for the things that happened in Germany, but in blaming Hitler for all the evils one is overlooking a considerable number of those who are truly responsible, people who are being allowed to pursue their course to similar ends all over again- nothing to stop them.

I do not claim to understand their motives. Perhaps a clergyman would. No one is forcing them to obey orders nowadays — they wouldn't obey them anyway — and still the pattern remains unchanged. Fascism and Nazism were solving the problems — with violence — and so were the psychiatrists.

The Nazis may have been disbanded, but the psychiatrists still linger on among us. Maybe this is the secret weapon Goebbels boasted about which would lead to the rebirth of the Reich — not a super-bomb and not a death ray, but a blueprint for a psychiatric slave state.

Bibliography

ALEXANDER, LEO, Neuropathology and Neurophysiology, including Electro-encephalography, in Wartime Germany. CIOS Item 24 File No XXVII-1 London (No date).

ALEXANDER, LEO, Public Mental Health Practices in Germany: Sterilization and Execution of Patients Suffering from Nervous or Mental Disease. CIOS Item 24 File No XXVIII-50. London (No date).

BAUR, E., FISCHER, E., and LENZ, F., Menschliche Erblichkeitslehre und Rassenhygiene. Band I: Menschliche Erblichkeitslehre. Band II: Menschliche Auslese und Rassenhygiene (Eugenik) Munchen 1927 and 1931.

BINDING, K, and HOCHE, A., Die Freigabe der Vernichtung Lebensunwerten Lebens. Leipzig, 1920.

BON, G., LE., Psychologie der Massen. 1908.

BUMKE, O., KOLB, G., ROEMER, H., and KAHN, E., (Herausgegeben) Handwörterbuch der Psychischen Hygiene und der Psychiatrischen Füsgorge. Berlin, 1931.

CARREL, A., Der Mensch das Unbekannte Wesen. Stuttgart.

CATEL, W., Grenzsituationen des Lebens. Nürnberg, 1962.

CHAMBERLAIN, H.S., Die Grundlagen des Neunzehnten Jahrhunderts. Munchen, 1B99.

DARWIN, C.R., Die Abstammung des Menschen und die Buchtwahl in Geschlechtlicher Beziehung. Leipzig, (No date) 18-?

DARWIN, C.R., Die Entstehung der Arten Durch Natürliche Zuchtwahl. Leipzig 18-?

DAS DEUTSCHE FUHRERLEXIKON 1934/1935. Berlin, 1934.

v. ECKARDT, M., and VILLINGER, W., (Herausgegeben). Gesundheit und Mitmenschliche Beziehungen (Bericht Ober die Internationale Tagung in Hiddesen bei Detmold 2-7 August 1951). Munchen, 1953.

EHRHARDT, H., Euthanasie und Vernichtung Lebensunwerten Lebens. Stuttgart 1965.

FEST, J., Das Gesicht des Dritten Reiches. Munchen, 1963.

FLUGEL, J.C., (Editor) International Congress on Mental Health, London, 1948 (4 volumes) London, 1948.

GOBINEAU, A., Versuch über die Unglsichheit der Menschenrassen. Stuttgart, 1898.

GOVERNMENT PRINTING OFFICE, Trials of War Criminals Before the Nuremberg Military Tribunals (Kriegsverbrecherprozesse vor den Nürnberger Militärgerichten) 13 Vols. Washington, 1951-1952.

GUTT, A., RÜDIN, E., and RUTTKE, F., Gesetz zur Verhütung Erbkranken Nachwuchses vom 14. Juli 1933. Munich, 1934.

HARSCH, J.C., Pattern for Conquest. London, 1942.

HILBERG, R., The Destruction of the European Jews. Chicago, 1961.

HITLER, Adolf. Mein Kampf. Munich, 1940.

HOFF, H., and ARNOLD, O.H., Germany and Austria. In Bellak, L., Contemporary European Psychiatry. New York, 1961.

HONOLKA, B., Die Kreuzeischreiber: Arzte ohne Gewissen. Euthanasie im Dritten Reich. Hamburg, 1961.

JOSIAH MACY, JR. FOUNDATION. Health and Human Relations in Germany. (Report of the Second Conference on Problems of Health and Human Relations in Germany. Held at the Williamsburg Lodge, Williamsburg, Virginia, U.S.A. December 10-15, 1950). New York.

JOSIAH MACY, JR. FOUNDATION. Health and Human Relations (Report of a Conference on Health and Human Relations Held at Hiddesen Near Detmold, Germany, August 2-7, 1951). New York, 1953.

KINTNER, E.W., (Editor) Trial of Alfons Klein, Adolf Wahlmann et al. (The Hadamar Trial). London, 1949.

KRAUSNICK, H., BUCHHEIM, H., BROSZAT, M., and JACOBSEN, H.A., Anatomie des SS-Staates. Olten und Freiburg im Breisgau, 1965.

LAPOUGE, V. DE, Der Arier und seine Bedeutung für die Gemeinschaft. Frankfurt a. M., 1939.

MALTHUS, T.R., Versuch über das Bevölkerungs-Gesetz. 1807 and 1964.

MASER, W., Hitler's Mein Kampf, 1966.

MITSCHERLICH, A., and MIELKE, F., Medizin ohne Menschlichkeit. Heidelberg, 1949.

PLATEN-HALLERMUND, A., Die Tötung Geisteskranker in Deutschland. Frankfurt, 1948.

PLOETZ, A., Grundlinien einer Rassenhygiene. Berlin, 1895.

REITLINGER, G., Die Endlösung. Berlin, 1956.

SEMMEL, B., Imperialism and Social Reform. London, 1960.

SHIRER, W.L., Berlin Diary. The Journal of a Foreign Correspondent 1934-1941. London, 1941.

SIMPSON, G.E., Darwin and Social Darwinism. In Clough, Gay and Warner, The European Past. N.Y., 1964.

SPENCER, H., Social Statics. N.Y., 1954.

STODARD, L., Into the Darkness. Nazi Germany Today. London, 1941.

TERNON, Y., and HELMAN, S., Histoire de la Médecine SS ou le Mythe du Racisme Biologique. Paris, 1969.

TERNON, Y., and HELMAN, S., Le Massacre des Aliénés. Paris, 1971.

WEINRICH, MAX. Hitler's Professors. New York, 1946.

WERTHAM, F., A Sign for Cain. London, 1966.

WILLIAMS, F.E., Proceedings of the First International Congress on Mental Hygiene (Held at Washington D.C., U.S.A. May 5th to 10th, 1930) 2 Vols. NY, 1932.

JOURNALS

Mental Health (UK)
Der Nervenarzt (G)
Zeitschrift für Psychische Hygiene (G)
Archiv für Rassen-und Gesellschaftsbiologie (G)
Eugenics Review (UK)

REPORTS AND ANNUAL REPORTS

Central Association for Mental Welfare (UK)
National Council for Mental Hygiene (UK)
Eugenics Education Society (UK)
Eugenics Society (UK)
National Association for Mental Health (UK)
Kaiser Wilhelm Gesellschaft (G)
Internationalen Federation Eugenischer Organisationen
International Committee for Mental Hygiene
World Federation for Mental Health

Appendix

States Having Sterilization Laws in 1956

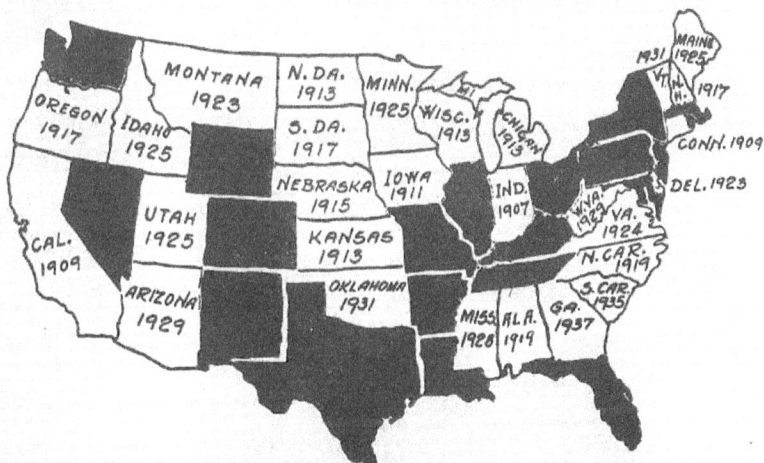

Date indicates the year in which a law was first passed; later revisions or amendments are not shown.

Sterilizations Reported

Per 100,000 Population[1]

1956

Georgia 7.22	New Hampshire 1.43	California .... .17
North Carolina 4.88	Indiana .... .86	West Virginia ...... .15
Delaware 2.98	Arizona .... .76	Maine .... .11
Virginia 2.38	Minnesota .... .59	Wisconsin .... .03
Iowa 2.26	Nebraska .... .56	Idaho 0
North Dakota 2.13	Michigan .... .36	Kansas 0
Oregon 1.98	Connecticut .... .31	Montana 0
Utah 1.84	South Dakota .... .29	Oklahoma 0
South Carolina 1.83	Mississippi .... .28	Vermont 0

Types of State Laws

STATE	Voluntary[1]	Compulsory[2]	Voluntary & Compulsory[3]	Extramural[4]	Eugenics Board[5]
*ALABAMA		x			
ARIZONA		x			
CALIFORNIA		x			
*CONNECTICUT		x			
DELAWARE		x		x	
*GEORGIA		x			x
*IDAHO		x		x	x
INDIANA		x			
*IOWA		x		x	x
*KANSAS		x			
*MAINE			x		
*MICHIGAN		x		x	
MINNESOTA	x			a	
MISSISSIPPI		x			
*MONTANA		x			x
*NEBRASKA		x			
NEW HAMPSHIRE		x			
*NORTH CAROLINA			x	x	x
*NORTH DAKOTA		x			
OKLAHOMA		x			
*OREGON		x		x	x
SOUTH CAROLINA		x			
*SOUTH DAKOTA			x	x	
UTAH		x		x	
VERMONT	x				
VIRGINIA		x			
WEST VIRGINIA		x			
WISCONSIN		x			

1. Consent of defective person, spouse or guardian required.
2. Consent of defective person not required.
3. Law contains provision for either voluntary or compulsory.
4. Law contains provision for individuals outside of institutions.
5. Authorization agency for sterilization operation. (Other states: operations passed on by designated state agencies.)

Sterilizations Reported in the United States to January 1, 1957

State	1956 Total	1955 Total	Grand Total — Total	Male	Female	Mentally Ill — Total	Male	Female	Cumulative Totals[1] — Mentally Deficient[1] Total	Male	Female	Others[2] — Total	Male	Female
Alabama[3]	8	1	224	129	95				224	129	95			
Arizona		25	30	10	20	24	10	14	6		6			
California	23	25	19,985	10,131	9,854	11,683	5,936	5,747	7,514	3,417	4,097	788	778	10
Connecticut	7	3	542	45	497	414	21	393	128	24	104			
Delaware	12		871	449	422	278	207	71	567	242	325	26		26
Georgia	268	261	2,490	1,023	1,467	1,855	786	1,069	626	237	389	9		9
Idaho	2	2	33	8	25	12	2	10	20	6	14	1		1
Indiana	34	94	2,325	1,148	1,177	609	302	307	1,712	845	867	4	1	3
Iowa	61	47	1,682	488	1,194	788	274	514	794	182	612	100	32	68
Kansas			3,025	1,763	1,262	2,063	1,210	853	849	511	338	113	42	71
Maine	1	26	305	44	261	21	6	15	214	38	176	70		70
Michigan	27	61	3,550	933	2,617	427	76	351	2,843	798	2,045	280	59	221
Minnesota	19	9	2,313	516	1,797	410	119	291	1,902	396	1,506	1	1	
Mississippi	6		602	154	448	530	140	390	58	14	44	14		14
Montana		15	256	72	184	42	17	25	214	55	159			
Nebraska	8	15	852	399	453	164	61	103	679	335	344	9	3	6
New Hampshire	8	4	670	148	522	246	27	219	372	121	251	52		52
New York[3]			42	1	41	41		41	1	1		1		1
North Carolina	216	289	4,472	937	3,535	1,334	379	955	2,826	481	2,345	312	77	235
North Dakota	14	16	961	352	609	379	128	251	546	211	335	36	13	23
Oklahoma		1	556	122	434	306	71	235	250	51	199			
Oregon	38	28	2,177	846	1,331	825	356	469	1,239	454	785	113	36	77
South Carolina	43	30	201	18	183	77	6	71	123	12	111	1		1
South Dakota	2	2	779	281	498	23	7	16	738	268	470	18	6	12
Utah	15	9	732	336	396	112	44	68	620	292	328			
Vermont			252	83	169	13	1	12	211	73	138	28	9	19
Virginia	87	111	6,683	2,640	4,043	3,415	1,320	2,095	3,113	1,238	1,875	155	82	73
Washington[3]		33	685	184	501	403	147	256	276	33	243	6	4	2
West Virginia	3		98	15	83	23	2	21	52	11	41	23	2	21
Wisconsin	1		1,793	392	1,401	8	5	3	1,784	386	1,398	1	1	
Totals	901	1,067	59,186	23,667	35,519	26,525	11,660	14,865	30,500	10,860	19,640	2,161	1,147	1,014

EUGENICS EDUCATION SOCIETY, 1916.

Elected President
MAJOR LEONARD DARWIN.

Nominated Hon. Secretaries
MRS. A. C. GOTTO, DR. E. SCHUSTER.

Nominated Hon. Treasurer
MR. VON FLEISCHL.

Elected Vice=Presidents
DR. RICHARD ARTHUR, M.L.A., President, New South Wales Branch
SIR JAMES BARR, President, Liverpool Branch.
DR. BENHAM, President, Dunedin Branch.
MR. H. W. BISHOP, S.M., President, Christchurch Branch.
SIR JAMES CRICHTON-BROWNE, F.R.S., Ex-President, 1908-9.
BISHOP D'ARCY, President, Belfast Branch.
PROFESSOR STARR JORDAN, President, Eugenic Section, American Genetic Association.
PROFESSOR H. B. KIRK, M.A., President, Wellington Branch.
MR. W. C. MARSHALL, M.A., President, Haslemere Branch.
THE RT. HON. LORD MOULTON, P.C., F.R.S., President, Birmingham Heredity Society.
MR. J. L. OTTER, J.P., President, Brighton Branch.
M. EDMOND PERRIER, President, Société Française D'Eugénique.
DR. A. PLOETZ, President, International Society for Race Hygiene.
PROFESSOR E. B. POULTON, F.R.S., President, Oxford Branch.
PROFESSOR SERGI, President, Comitato Italiano per gli Studi di Eugenica.
PROFESSOR SEWARD, F.R.S., President, Cambridge Eugenics Society.
BISHOP WELLDON, President, Manchester Branch.

Hon. Members
THE RT. HON. A. J. BALFOUR, P.C.
SIR ARCHIBALD GEIKIE, F.R.S.
HER GRACE, THE DUCHESS OF MARLBOROUGH.

Elected Members of Council

LADY BARRETT.
MR. CROFTON BLACK.
SIR E. BRABROOK, C.B.
MRS. THEODORE CHAMBERS.
HON. SIR JOHN COCKBURN, K.C.M.G.
MISS E. CORRY.
MR. R. NEWTON CRANE.
MR. A. E. CRAWLEY.
SIR H. CUNNINGHAM, K.C.I.E.
DR. LANGDON DOWN.
MR. HAVELOCK ELLIS.
PROFESSOR J. FINDLAY.
MR. E. G. WHELER GALTON.
DR. GREENWOOD.
DR. W. HADLEY.
MRS. HENDERSON.
COLONEL HILLS, F.R.S.
VERY REV. W. R. INGE, D.D., Dean of St. Paul's.
MISS KIRBY.

MR. ERNEST LANE, F.R.C.S.
PROFESSOR MACBRIDE.
LADY OWEN MACKENZIE.
MR. ROBERT MOND.
DR. F. W. MOTT, F.R.S.
MR. G. P. MUDGE.
MRS. G. POOLEY.
DR. ARCHDALL REID.
MR. JOHN RUSSELL.
MR. F. C. S. SCHILLER, D.Sc.
PROFESSOR A. SCHUSTER, F.R.S.
MR. EDGAR SCHUSTER, D.Sc.
DR. C. G. SELIGMAN.
PROFESSOR SPEARMAN.
PROFESSOR J. A. THOMSON.
DR. A. F. TREDGOLD.
MRS. ALEC TWEEDIE.
MR. W. C. D. WHETHAM, F.R.S.
DR. DOUGLAS WHITE.

BELFAST.
PROFESSOR J. A. LINDSAY.

BIRMINGHAM.
MR. CARY GILSON.
MR. HUMPHREY HUMPHREYS.
MR. P. MILLS.

BRIGHTON.
MR. A. J. HALL.

HASLEMERE.
MR. W. C. MARSHALL.

LIVERPOOL.
MR. R. T. BODEY.
MR. R. D. LAURIE.
ALDERMAN T. R. BULLEY.

MANCHESTER.
DR. MUMFORD.

NEW SOUTH WALES.
(To be appointed.)

NEW ZEALAND.
Dunedin, Christchurch, Wellington.
HON. T. A. MACKENZIE.
(High Commissioner).

OXFORD.
MR. E. SCHUSTER, D.Sc.

The Board of the English Eugenics Education Society 1915-1916. Ploetz was an elected Vice-President.

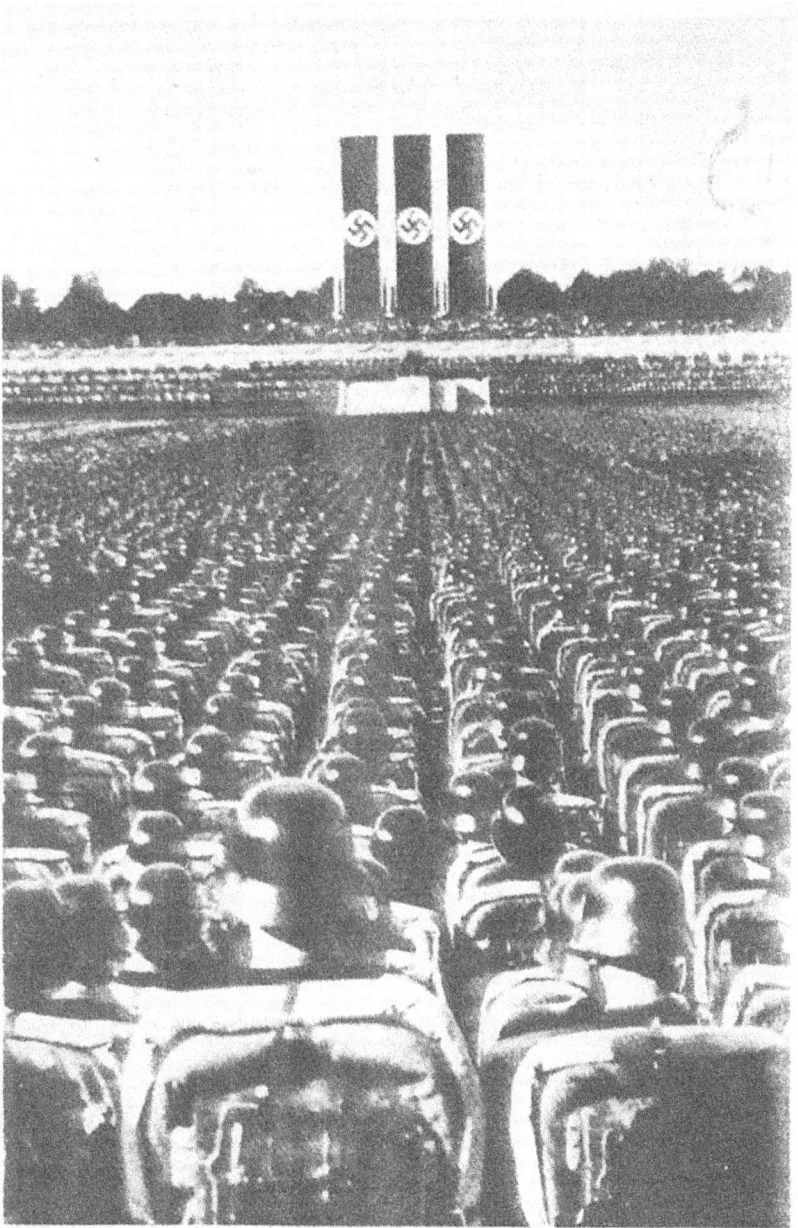

Nuremberg rally. How many of these people later served as guards in the eugenic death camps?

Gesetz zur Verhütung erbkranken Nachwuchses

vom 14. Juli 1933
nebst Ausführungsverordnungen

Bearbeitet und erläutert von

Dr. med. Arthur Gütt
Ministerialdirektor
im Reichsministerium des Innern

Dr. med. Ernst Rüdin
o. ö. Professor für Psychiatrie an der Universität und Direktor
des Kaiser Wilhelm-Instituts für Genealogie und Demographie
der Deutschen Forschungsanstalt für Psychiatrie in München

Dr. jur. Falk Ruttke
Geschäftsführender Direktor des Reichsausschusses für Volksgesundheitsdienst
beim Reichsministerium des Innern

Mit Beiträgen:

Die Eingriffe zur Unfruchtbarmachung des Mannes und zur Entmannung.

Von Geheimrat Prof. Dr. med. Erich Lexer, München .

Die Eingriffe zur Unfruchtbarmachung der Frau.

Von Prof. Dr. med. Heinrich Eymer, München

Mit 26 zum Teil farbigen Abbildungen

Zweite, neubearbeitete Auflage

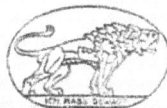

J. F. Lehmanns Verlag / München 1936

Two months after the Nazi seizure of power, the racial hygienists show their hand.

88

Menschliche Erblichkeitslehre und Rassenhygiene

von

Prof. Dr. E. Baur, Prof. Dr. E. Fischer
und Prof. Dr. F. Lenz

Band I:
Menschliche Erblichkeitslehre

Band II:
Menschliche Auslese und Rassenhygiene (Eugenik)

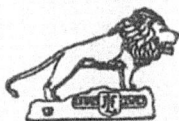

J. F. LEHMANNS VERLAG / MÜNCHEN 1932

49. *Schuster, E.*, E u g e n i c s, London and Glasgow 1913. (264 S.)
50. *Siemens, H. W.*, V e r e r b u n g s l e h r e, R a s s e n h y g i e n e u n d B e-
v ö l k e r u n g s p o l i t i k. 4. Aufl. Lehmann, München 1930. (147 S.,
oktav.)
51. *Stoddard, L.*, The Revolt against Civilization. New York 1922. Deutsche
Übersetzung: D e r K u l t u r u m s t u r z. D i e D r o h u n g d e s U n t e r-
m e n s c h e n. München 1925. (212 S., gemeinverständliche, packende
Werbeschrift.)
52. *Wiggam, A. E.*, T h e n e x t A g e o f M a n. Indianapolis 1927. (418 S.)

II. Bücher zum ersten Abschnitt des zweiten Bandes.

53. *Ammon, O.*, D i e n a t ü r l i c h e A u s l e s e b e i m M e n s c h e n. Jena
1893. (326 S.)
54. — — D i e G e s e l l s c h a f t s o r d n u n g u n d i h r e n a t ü r l i c h e n
G r u n d l a g e n. 1. Aufl. 1895, 3. Aufl. 1910. (262 S. Historisch bedeutsames Werk über die soziale Auslese.)
55. *Carr- Saunders, A. M.*, T h e P o p u l a t i o n P r o b l e m. Oxford 1922.
(516 S., mit sehr vielem historischen und ethnologischen Material.)
56. — — P o p u l a t i o n. London 1925. (111 S., oktav.)
57. *Darré, R. W.*, D a s B a u e r n t u m a l s L e b e n s q u e l l d e r n o r d i-
s c h e n R a s s e. Lehmann, München 1929. (482 S.)
58. *Elster, A.*, S o z i a l b i o l o g i e. Bevölkerungswissenschaft und Gesell-
schaftshygiene. Berlin u. Leipzig 1923. (483 S.; in mancher Hinsicht anfechtbar, enthält aber wertvolles Material.)
59. *Gobineau, J. A. Graf von*, V e r s u c h ü b e r d i e U n g l e i c h h e i t d e r
M e n s c h e n r a s s e n. Deutsche Übersetzung von L. S c h e m a n n, Stuttgart 1898. (1853—55 erschienenes Werk, von historischer Bedeutung.)
60. *Grant, M.*, T h e P a s s i n g o f t h e G r e a t R a c e. 2. Aufl. New York
1918. (296 S.; deutsche Übersetzung: „Der Untergang der großen
Rasse", München 1925; modernes amerikanisches Werk im Geiste Go-
bineaus.)
61. *Günther, H. F. K.*, R a s s e n k u n d e d e s d e u t s c h e n V o l k e s.
12. Aufl. München 1928 (509 S., behandelt auch die Auslesevorgänge.)
62. — — R a s s e n g e s c h i c h t e d e s h e l l e n i s c h e n u n d d e s r ö m i-
s c h e n V o l k e s. München 1929. (130 S.).
63. — — R a s s e n k u n d e d e s j ü d i s c h e n V o l k e s. Lehmann, München
1930. (352 S.).
64. *Hartnacke, W.*, N a t u r g r e n z e n g e i s t i g e r B i l d u n g. Leipzig 1930.
(212 S., enthält wertvolles Material über soziale Auslese.)
65. *Just, G.*, V e r e r b u n g u n d E r z i e h u n g. Berlin 1930. (233 S., mit
Beiträgen von 7 Mitarbeitern, in Einzelheiten anfechtbar, im ganzen
aber wertvoll.)
66. *de Lapouge, V.*, L e s s é l e c t i o n s s o c i a l e s. Paris 1896. (503 S.).
67. *Marcuse, M.*, D e r e h e l i c h e P r ä v e n t i v v e r k e h r, s e i n e V e r-
b r e i t u n g, V e r u r s a c h u n g u n d M e t h o d i k, d a r g e s t e l l t u n d
b e l e u c h t e t a n 3 0 0 E h e n. Stuttgart 1917.
68. *Niceforo, A.*, A n t h r o p o l o g i e d e r n i c h t b e s i t z e n d e n K l a s s e n.
Deutsche Übersetzung Leipzig 1910. (Bedeutsames Werk zur sozialen
Auslese mit wichtigem Originalmaterial.)

*Professor Lenz bases his work on the "scientific" works of such
authorities: Stoddard, American racist; Ammon, German racist;
Darré, later Nazi Minister of Agriculture; Gobineau, French racist;
Grant, American racist: Günther, crude German racist; de Lapouge,
French racist and racial hygienist.*

r Entwicklung des Deutschen Reichs seit der Machtübernahme unseres Führers am 30. Januar 1933.

Es kann sich in dieser kurzen Übersicht, die hauptsächlich für unsere sländischen Leser bestimmt ist, nur darum handeln, auf die wichtigsten rtschritte hinzuweisen, die direkt oder indirekt auf unserem Gebiet der ssen- und Gesellschaftsbiologie sowie der Rassen- und Gesellschaftsgiene erfolgt sind, einem Gebiet, das von Adolf Hitler als die wichtigste undlage unseres völkischen und staatlichen Lebens hingestellt worden ist. Die Reformen begannen mit dem Erlaß des Gesetzes zur Verhütung bkranken Nachwuchses vom 14. Juli 1933. Nach diesem Gesetz kann, r erbkrank ist, durch chirurgischen Eingriff oder andere Verfahren unchtbar gemacht (sterilisiert) werden, wenn nach den Erfahrungen der tlichen Wissenschaft mit großer Wahrscheinlichkeit zu erwarten ist, daß ne Nachkommen an schweren körperlichen oder geistigen Erbschäden den werden.

Dem vorstehenden Gesetz folgte das Gesetz zum Schutze des deuthen Blutes und der deutschen Ehre vom 15. September 1935. Darch wurden Eheschließungen und außerehelicher Verkehr zwischen Jun und Staatsangehörigen deutschen oder artverwandten Blutes verboten. Ferner folgte das Gesetz zum Schutz der Erbgesundheit des deutnen Volkes (das Ehegesundheitsgesetz) vom 18. Oktober 1935, wonach e Ehe nicht geschlossen werden darf, wenn einer der Verlobten an einer t Ansteckungsgefahr verbundenen Krankheit leidet, die eine erhebliche hädigung der Gesundheit des anderen Teiles oder der Nachkommen bechten läßt; wenn einer der Verlobten entmündigt ist oder unter vorläuer Vormundschaft steht; wenn einer der Verlobten, ohne entmündigt zu n, an einer geistigen Störung leidet, die die Ehe für die Volksgemeinaft unerwünscht erscheinen läßt, und wenn einer der Verlobten an einer bkrankheit im Sinne des Gesetzes zur Verhütung erbkranken Nachwuch-leidet. Vor der Eheschließung haben die Verlobten durch ein Zeugnis des sundheitsamtes nachzuweisen, daß ein Ehehindernis im Sinne des Gezes nicht vorliegt.

Alle diese Gesetze sind durch Nachträge, Verordnungen und Kommen-e in ihrer sorgfältigen Durchführung erleichtert und ermöglicht worden d haben Ströme von wohltätigen Wirkungen aus ihrer Anwendung im lk aus sich hervorgehen lassen, Wirkungen, die sich in ihrer vollen Kraft t in der nahen und besonders in der fernen Zukunft entfalten werden.

Weitere rassenhygienische Maßnahmen waren die zahlreichen Ehestands-darlehen und Kinderbeihilfen in den Familien besonders der Kinderreichen, die zu einer bedeutenden Erhöhung der in starkem Rückgang gewesenen deutschen Geburtenziffer führten.

Die Erziehung der deutschen Jugend in geistiger, seelischer und körperlicher Beziehung wurde und wird weiter in steigendem Maße un-abhängig von konfessioneller und fremdrassiger Leitung durchgeführt und dem Staate unterstellt. Dadurch werden das Wachsen und die Erhaltung des nationalsozialistischen Geistes, die schon ohnehin durch staatliche und parteiliche Organisation weitgehend beeinflußt sind, dauernd sichergestellt.

Der unser Kultur- und staatliches Leben so stark beeinflussende, ja viel-fach beherrschende jüdische Bevölkerungsteil wurde stark zurück-gedrängt, so in der Wehrmacht, in der Wirtschaft, im Richterstande, bei den Lehrern aller Arten und Stufen, in der Presse, im Theater, im Film.

Die schwer auf unserem Volke lastende Arbeitslosigkeit wurde bis auf relativ geringe Reste heruntergesetzt und die Lage der arbeitenden Klassen überhaupt in gesundheitlicher, wirtschaftlicher und sozialer Be-ziehung stark gehoben.

Die Sicherung unseres Volkes bei seiner rasslichen Aufwärtsbewegung wurde weiter bewirkt durch den Austritt aus dem Völkerbunde, die kühne Null- und Nichtigerklärung der Verträge von Versailles und St. Germain, Schritte, die starke Schutzmaßnahmen für das Deutsche Reich ermöglichten, wie die Schaffung einer großen modernen Wehrmacht, wie die entschlossene Besetzung des Rheinlandes durch Einmarsch deutscher Truppen, wie die deutsch-japanisch-italienische Eini-gung gegen den Kommunismus und die Schaffung der „Achse" Deut-sches Reich–Italien und wie schließlich die wunderbare Wiederver-einigung Österreichs mit dem Deutschen Reich, die nicht nur einen starken Zuwachs an militärischen, wirtschaftlichen und kulturellen Mög-lichkeiten bedeutete, sondern vor allem die alte Sehnsucht der Deutschen im Reich und in Österreich verwirklichte, für immer und alle Zeiten zu einem Großdeutschland zusammenzuschmelzen.

Dieses einige Hauptteile des gewaltigen Werkes unseres Führers und seiner Getreuen!

Hitler rückt durch seine Taten in die Reihe unserer größten Führer seit den ältesten Zeiten!

Unser Volk hat das erkannt und hängt ihm mit dankbarem Herzen an. Kein deutscher Fürst, kein deutscher König oder Kaiser ist jemals von seinem ganzen Volke so leidenschaftlich geliebt worden wie Adolf Hitler.

Alfred Ploetz.   Ernst Rüdin.

Archiv für Rassenhygiene.

On the Development of the Third Reich since the Seizure of Power by our Führer on January the 30th 1933.

This short synopsis which is directed mainly at our foreign reader can only serve the purpose of pointing out the most important advances directly or indirectly concernnig our areas of Racial and Social Biology and Racial and Social Hygiene. These are areas which Adolf Hitler has pointed out to be the most important foundations of our racial and state life.

The reforms began with the passage of the law for "The Prevention of Hereditarily Ill Descendants" on the 14th of July 1933. According to this law, anyone who is hereditarily ill can be made barren (sterilised) when in the view of medical science it could be expected on a high probability that his descendants would suffer from grievous physical and mental hereditary defects.

This was followed by "The Law for the Protection of German Blood and German Honour" on the 15th of September 1935. By this all marriages and extra marital relationships between Jews and citizens of German stock or related stock was forbidden.

This was followed by the "Law for the Protection of Hereditary Health" of the German People (The Marriage Health Law) on the 18th of October 1935 whereby a marriage could not be undertaken if one of the betrothed is suffering from a contagious illness whereby severe damage to the health of the other party is to be feared. Also when one of the betrothed couple has been incapacitated or is under tutelage, or when one of the betrothed couple without being incapacitated suffers from a mental defect, which makes the marriage undesirable for the racial community and when one of the betrothed suffers from a hereditary disease by the definitions given in the "Law for The Prevention of Hereditarily Ill descendants." Before undertaking the marriage the couple must prove by attestation of the Health Office, that no reason exists for the prevention of the marriage under law.

The diligent enforcement of these laws has been made easier and more possible through supplements, regulations and commentaries, and their application has caused many beneficial results for the populace, results whose full effect will be felt in the future.

Further racial hygienic measures were the marriage loans and child support laws especially for families with many children.

These have led to an increase of the birthrate which was declining strongly.

The education of German Youth in mental, spiritual and physical respects is being undertaken more and more independently of religion and alien racial influence, and is more under the control of the state. This ensures the growth and the preservation of the national-socialist spirit, which is already influenced to a great degree by state and party organisations.

The Jewish part of the population which influences our cultural life so strongly, and often even controls it, has been driven back strongly in the Wehrmacht, in the economy, in the judiciary, among teachers of all kinds and levels, in the press, in the theatre and in the film industry.

Unemployment which was burdening our race so heavily has been done away with except for relatively small sections, and the position of the working classes especially as regards health, economy and social services has been greatly improved.

The safeguarding of our race in its racial progress was further assisted by the withdrawal from the League of Nations and the daring declaration that made null and void the Treaties of Versailles and of St. Germain, steps which made strong protective measures possible for the German Reich such as the creation of a large modern Wehrmacht, the resolute occupation of the Rhineland by German troops, the German - Japanese - Italian unification against Communism and the creation of the "Axis" German Reich - Italy and finally the wonderful reunification of Austria with the German Reich. This brought about not only an increase of military, economic and cultural possibilities, but above all it realised the old desire of the Germans in the Reich and in Austria to be united for all times in a Greater Germany.

These are some of the major points of the stupendous achievements of our Führer and his faithful followers !

Through his deeds Hitler moves up into the ranks of our greatest leaders since oldest times !

Our people have realised this and are devoted to him with grateful hearts. No German prince, no German king or emperor has ever been loved so passionately by his whole people as Adolf Hitler.

Alfred Ploetz   Ernst Rüdin.

Rüdin and Ploetz speak for themselves. No comment.

Zu Adolf Hitlers Geburtstag.

Am 20. April wird unser Führer 49 Jahre alt, zehn Tage nach einer Volksabstimmung im alten Reich und Österreich, die ihm die unerhörte Zahl von über 99 Ja-Stimmen auf das Hundert abgegebener Stimmen brachte.

Jeder, der die Begeisterung unseres Volkes miterlebt hat oder der die Berichte seiner Freunde im alten Reich und Österreich darüber hörte, weiß, daß die gehässigen und verdächtigenden Stimmen über die Ehrlichkeit des Wahlaktes in das Reich grauer Fabel gehören. Wenn je unser Volk (bis auf kleinste Reste) vollkommen einig war, war das diesmal der Fall.

Wir wünschen Adolf Hitler aus tiefem Herzen, daß es ihm vom Schicksal vergönnt sein möge, Großdeutschland weiter zu den lichten Höhen friedlicher Entwicklung zu führen!

Alfred Ploetz.   Ernst Rüdin.

On the Occasion of Adolf Hitler's Birthday.

On the 20th of April our Führer will be 49 years old, ten days after a plebiscite in the old Reich and in Austria which brought him the unheard of figure of 99 out of a hundred votes.

Anyone who has been involved in the enthusiasm of our people or who heard the reports of his friends in the old Reich and in Austria knows that the hateful and suspicious doubts raised about the honesty of the polling belong to the realm of the grey fable. If ever our people were unanimous (except for minor sectors), then this is the time.

We wish for Adolf Hitler from the depth of our hearts that fate may grant he keep leading Greater Germany to the bright heights of peaceful development!

Alfred Ploetz   Ernst Rüdin.

Rüdin and Ploetz congratulate their Führer from the depth of their hearts.

Notizen

Der uns aufgezwungene Krieg und die Rassenhygiene.

Ein moderner Krieg, ob siegreich bestanden oder nicht, bedeutet, wie jeder Rassenhygieniker weiß, für alle betroffenen Nationen eine furchtbare Gegenauslese, die Vernichtung einer Blüte von gerade besonders tüchtigen jungen Menschen im Beginn der Fortpflanzungszeit. Durch diesen Massentod fällt nicht bloß die an ihre eigene Person geknüpfte Kulturleistung fort, sondern auch ihre gesamte Nachkommenschaft, welche sie ohne Krieg gezeugt hätte. Diesem nur sehr schwer wieder gutzumachenden Schaden gegenüber kommt als Nutzen für das Erbgut der Rasse die selektorische Ausmerze minderwertiger Anlagen in einem modernen Kriege sehr viel weniger, und heute sehr viel weniger als je, in Betracht. Denn die mit Hunger und Seuchen, d. h. mit stark selektorisch ausmerzend wirkenden, Kranke und organisch mangelhaft Veranlagte besonders hart treffenden Faktoren einhergehenden Kriege sind sehr viel seltener geworden, da heute Hygiene und Lebensmittelverteilungs-Organisation bei den meisten Kulturnationen so vollendet arbeiten, daß erblich defekte und krank Veranlagte gegenüber den Normalen in heutigen Kriegen wohl nicht mehr so stark benachteiligt sein dürften wie in früheren.

So wird also die rassenhygiene-feindliche Wirkung eines modernen Krieges heute nur noch verstärkt.

Man sollte meinen, daß solche für das Blühen der Kulturvölker auch in der Zukunft maßgebenden Überlegungen den gegenwärtigen Krieg hätten verhindern sollen. Die deutschen Rassenhygieniker haben denn auch seit Jahrzehnten und seit der Gründung des Dritten Reiches in verstärktem Maße gegenüber den anderen Kulturnationen und insbesondere auch gegenüber England und Frankreich keinen Zweifel darüber gelassen, daß ein Krieg zwischen ihnen neben allen anderen Schrecken immer auch einen gegenseitigen rassenhygienischen Vernichtungskampf bedeuten würde, und daß daher der Friede, ein friedliches Zusammenarbeiten, ja wir können auch ruhig sagen, ein friedlicher fruchtbarer Wettbewerb im Interesse aller kulturell schöpferischen und verwandten Völker liege. Auch die deutschen Gelehrten überhaupt, die Politiker, die Staatsmänner, ließen es in diplomatischen Verhandlungen, in Wirtschafts- und Handelskonferenzen, in internationalen wissenschaftlichen und anderen Vereinigungen und Kongressen an keinen Vorschlägen und immer wieder unermüdlich angesetzten Versuchen fehlen, eine friedliche Zusammenarbeit sicherzustellen.

Ein grausames Geschick hat es nicht zugelassen, diese Bemühungen mit Erfolg zu krönen: den allein unheilschwangere Fehlsteuerung eines Teils der europäischen Kulturpolitik hat es gewollt, daß verhältnismäßig dünne, aber mächtige und rücksichtslose Schichten des englischen und französischen Volkes in, wie es sich gezeigt hat, unüberwindlicher Eifersucht auf den Freiheits- und Unabhängigkeitsdrang des deutschen Volkes und in unerschütterlicher Absicht die völlige Hegemonie über das deutsche Volk wieder zu erringen und zu verstärken bis zur völligen militärischen, politischen, wirtschaftlichen und finanziellen Ohnmacht Deutschlands.

Anfangs wurde von diesen Schichten dem deutschen Freiheitsdrang noch das berüchtigte Heuchel-Argument des „Kampfes für die Freiheit der kleinen Völker" entgegengesetzt. Auch die abgegriffenen täglich und stündlich als natur-unwahr erwiesene französische Revolutionsparole der Freiheit, Gleichheit und Brüderlichkeit unter allen Menschen sollte die jedem Denkenden und Geschichtskundigen klar erwiesenen,

So gibt es für das nationalsozialistisch geeinte und durchorganisierte Deutschland nur eines: den ihm von Englands kriegsinteressierten Schichten und Juden und seinen entsprechenden französischen Trabantenschichten aufgezwungenen und feierlich angesagten Krieg auch mit Krieg zu beantworten. In Deutschland, das von dem zielbewußten Freiheitswillen seines Führers geleitet und das ihm in allen seinen Schichten in diesem Ringen bis zum Sieg die Treue halten wird, gibt es heute nur ein gemeinsames Ziel: Kampf gegen den uns aufgezwungenen Krieg bis zur absoluten Sicherung unserer Freiheit und unseres Lebensraumes. Gewiß, wir denken nach wie vor rassenhygienisch, weil wir das ewige Deutschland wollen. Deshalb wollen und müssen wir als Freie siegen und weiterleben! Dann auch werden wir, das ist unsere feste Zuversicht, im Frieden die Schäden des Krieges durch um so folgerichtigere Rassenhygiene in unserem Volke wieder gut machen können.

Ploetz.   Rüdin.

The War Forced Upon Us and Racial Hygiene.

A modern war whether carried out victoriously or not, brings about, as every racial hygienist knows, the horrible contra-selection, and destruction of the flower of youth at the beginning of its reproductive period. This mass-death causes not only the loss of the individual's cultural achievements [but also the potential of all his descendants]. This damage, which can be rectified only through efforts, is balanced only slightly, by the selective elimination of inferior types, which improves the hereditary mass of the race. Wars where hunger and disease, as strong selective factors, have eliminated the severely ill and the organically defective, are things of the past. For in today's war hygiene and food distribution organisations in most of the civilized nations are so perfected that the genetically deficient and ill are not as severely handicapped as in earlier ones.

The counter-selective effects of a modern war are only strength-ened today.

One would think that such decisive considerations concerning the future of civilized races would have prevented the present war. For decades and especially since the foundation of the Third Reich, German racial hygienists have never left any doubt in the minds of other cultured nations and above all England and France, that a war between them would encompass, apart from all other horrors, a mutual racial extermination. For this reason, peace, a peaceful cooperation — yes we can go so far as to say a peaceful productive competition of all culturally creative and related peoples — would be in their interest. Even German scientists, politicians and statesmen have never failed to point out their ideas in their diplomatic negotiations, in economic and trade conferences, in international scientific and other meetings and congresses, and made attempts again and again to ensure peaceful cooperation.

A cruel fate has disallowed their success. Disastrous misguid-ance by a section of European politics has created a relatively small but powerful and ruthless stratum of English and French people who are jealous of the efforts to achieve freedom and liberty for the German People. They have come to power with the imperturbable intention of regaining full hegemony over the German People again and to strengthen it to a point of total military, political, economic and financial unconsciousness in Germany.

But the national socialistically united and thoroughly organised Germany will answer the war forced upon it and solemnly declared on it by the English warlike classes and Jews and the corresponding French classes. In Germany, led by the purposeful urge towards freedom of its Führer and in which all its classes will remain faithful in this struggle for victory, there is but one common goal: Fight the war forced upon us to the point of absolute security of our territory. Certainly, we still think in terms of racial hygiene because we want an eternal Germany. Therefore we will win as free people and will continue to live as such. Then, and this is our firm hope, we will be able to make good the damages of war to our people, through an even more consistent policy of racial hygiene, in peace.

PLOETZ   RUDIN

Rüdin and Ploetz once again.

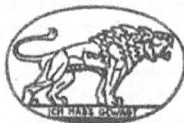

Archiv für
Rassen- und Gesellschaftsbiologie

einschließlich Rassen- und Gesellschaftshygiene

Zeitschrift

für die Erforschung des Wesens von Rasse und Gesellschaft und ihres gegenseitigen Verhältnisses, für die biologischen Bedingungen ihrer Erhaltung und Entwicklung sowie für die grundlegenden Probleme der Entwicklungslehre

Wissenschaftliches Organ
der Deutschen Gesellschaft für Rassenhygiene und des
Reichsausschusses für Volksgesundheitsdienst

Gegründet von

Prof., Dr. med., Dr. phil. h. c. Alfred Ploetz †

Herausgeber: Dr. med. Agnes Bluhm, Professor der Statistik und Bevölkerungspolitik Dr. F. Burgdörfer, Professor der Anthropologie Dr. E. Fischer, Professor Dr. W. Groß, Leiter des Rassenpolitischen Amtes der NSDAP, Staatssekretär a. D. ᛋᛋ-Brigadeführer Dr. med. A. Gütt, Professor für Allgemeine Biologie und menschliche Abstammungslehre Dr. G. Heberer, Professor der Rassenhygiene Dr. F. Lenz, Professor der Anthropologie Dr. Th. Mollison, Dr. jur. A. Nordenholz, Professor der Hygiene Dr. E. Rodenwaldt, Professor der Psychiatrie und der Rassenhygiene Dr. E. Rüdin, Professor für Rasse und Recht Oberregierungsrat Dr. F. Ruttke, Professor für arische Kultur und Sprachwissenschaft Dr. Walther Wüst

Schriftleitung

Prof. Dr. Ernst Rüdin, München

36. Band

J. F. Lehmanns Verlag, München-Berlin

The "high society" of racial hygiene: NSDAP and SS. Rüdin and his colleagues move in the best circles.

Die Vollendung Großdeutschlands

Als im März vorigen Jahres Österreich mit dem deutschen Altreich ver einigt wurde, ahnten wohl nur wenige, daß die Vereinigung des Sudeten landes mit dem neuen Reich nahe bevorstand und das wahre Großdeutsch land vollenden würde.

Trotz der bedeutend größeren politischen und militärischen Schwie rigkeiten gelang die Einfügung der deutschvölkischen Teile der Tscheche in das Deutsche Reich in der verhältnismäßig kurzen Zeit von weniger Monaten ohne nennenswerte Verluste der zivilen Bevölkerung und der ein marschierenden Teile des deutschen Heeres. Bei der Abstimmung lautete über 98% der abgegebenen Stimmen für den Anschluß.

Großdeutschland hatte nunmehr außer den 6½ Millionen Österreichern weitere 2½ Millionen Deutsche gewonnen, so daß der eigentliche völkische Block des neuen Reiches nunmehr nahezu 80 Millionen Volksgenossen zählt. Die militärischen, wirtschaftlichen und kulturellen Gewinne liegen auf der Hand, ebenso, was von unserem Standpunkt, den wir hier zu ver treten haben, äußerst wichtig ist, die direkten und indirekten Vorteile auf dem rassenhygienischen Gebiet.

Wiederum hat, wie der Erfolg lehrt, unser Führer mit unbeirrbarem staatsmännischem Blick Zeit und Ort der politischen Aktion und das Zu sammenspiel mit seinen Getreuen so sicher gelenkt, daß alles, was wir im April vorigen Jahres über ihn und sein gewaltiges Werk sagten, nun in womöglich noch verstärktem Maße gilt:

„Hitler rückt durch seine Taten in die Reihe unserer größten Führer seit den ältesten Zeiten! Unser Volk hat das erkannt und hängt ihm mit dankbarem Herzen an. Kein deutscher Fürst, kein deutscher König oder Kaiser ist jemals von seinem ganzen Volke so leidenschaftlich geliebt worden wie Adolf Hitler"[1].

Alfred Ploetz   Ernst Rüdin

---

[1] Archiv 1938, Heft 2, S. 186.

The Perfection of Great Germany

When in March last year, Austria was united with the German Old Reich, few anticipated that the reunion of the Sudetenland with the new Reich was forthcoming, and the true Great Germany would be completed.

In spite of the greater political and military difficulties, the integration of the German sections of Czechoslovakia into the German Reich succeeded in the relatively short time of a few months. There were no losses worth mentioning, to the civil population or the advancing German army. Over 98 % of the votes cast were for the annexation.

Apart from the 6 1/2 million Austrians, Great Germany has now won an additional 2 1/2 million Germans, and now the actual racial block of the Reich counts almost 80 million racial comrades. The military, economic and cultural gains are evident, just as the direct and indirect advantages are in the field of racial hygiene.

Again, as success shows our Führer has set with an unerring statesmanlike view the time and place of political action and staged the interplay of his faithful followers so surely, that everything we said about his tremendous deeds in April last year is now even more valid:

Through his deeds Hitler moves into the ranks of our greatest leaders since oldest times! Our people have realised this and are devoted to him with grateful hearts. No German prince, no German king or emperor has ever been loved so passionately by his whole people as Adolf Hitler.

Alfred Ploetz   Ernst Rüdin

Rüdin and Ploetz praise Hitler as the greatest Führer since the oldest times.

Aufgaben und Ziele der Deutschen Gesellschaft für Rassenhygiene.

Von Prof. Ernst Rüdin.

Die Gründung der Deutschen Gesellschaft für Rassenhygiene geht zurück auf das Jahr 1905, als Alfred Ploetz, der Begründer der deutschen Rassenhygiene und heute Ehrenmitglied der Gesellschaft, zusammen mit wenigen Freunden, zu denen auch ich gehörte, den ersten Versuch in Deutschland wagte, den rassenhygienischen Gedanken durch eine Vereinsorganisation weitere Verbreitung zu verschaffen. Aber trotz unserer beständigen Anstrengungen, die Öffentlichkeit darauf aufmerksam zu machen, daß endlich auch für die Rasse etwas zu geschehen habe, trotz unserer Hinweise schon am Anfang dieses Jahrhunderts, auf den kulturschöpferischen Wert der nordischen Rasse, auf die ungeheure Gefahr des Sinkens der deutschen Geburtenrate und auf die naturwidrige Aufpäppelung alles Erbschwachen, Kranken und Minderwertigen, konnten unsere Ideen keine Anerkennung bei den maßgebenden Stellen erzielen. Wenn es unserer geistigen Bewegung auch gelang, im Stillen und ganz allmählich die Köpfe und Herzen unserer besten Deutschen zu gewinnen, so sorgten doch die bekannten damals herrschenden Strömungen dafür, daß keine rassenhygienischen Maßnahmen getroffen werden durften. Die Bedeutung der Rassenhygiene ist in Deutschland erst durch das politische Werk Adolf Hitlers allen aufgeweckten Deutschen offenbar geworden, und erst durch ihn wurde endlich unser mehr als dreißigjähriger Traum zur Wirklichkeit, Rassenhygiene in die Tat umsetzen zu können.

Die gegenwärtige Kundgebung soll darum unserm Führer den tiefen Dank dafür vor aller Welt zum Ausdruck bringen.

Heute ist die Bahn für Rassenhygiene frei. Allein wir haben gerade nur die ersten Schrittchen auf ihr gemacht und es sind noch viele, viele Schritte zu gehen bis wesentliche Ziele der Rassenhygiene erreicht sind. Rassenhygiene ist keine Modesache, sondern sie muß ein Volk ständig begleiten, damit es immer auf der Höhe bleibt. Und diesen Weg unseres Volkes, unserer Rasse in die Zukunft nach rassenhygienischen Gesichtspunkten zu organisieren, das Volk mit all dem Rüstwerk, all dem geistigen und moralischen Proviant zu versehen, den es für seine schicksalsbestimmende Reise braucht, ist, im Verein mit anderen Organisationen und mit der Gesetzgebung, die Aufgabe der Deutschen Gesellschaft für Rassenhygiene, die durch das Verdienst des Herrn Reichsministers Dr. Frick im völkischen Sinne neu organisiert dasteht.

Duties and Aims of the German Society for Racial Hygiene
By Prof. Ernst Rüdin

The foundation of the German Society for Racial Hygiene was back in the year 1905, when Alfred Ploetz, the founder of German racial hygiene and today honorary member of the Society, together with a group of friends, to which I also belonged, undertook the first attempt in Germany to create a spread of the principles of racial Hygiene through the organisation of societies. Inspite of our constant endeavours to inform the public that it was about time that something was done about the race, in spite of our references even at the beginning of this century to the cultural-creative value of the Nordic race and the drastic danger of the decline of the German birthrate and the spoonfeeding of all hereditarily weak, ill and less valuable, which is contrary to nature, our ideas could find no recognition in authoritative positions. Even if our movement succeeded in silently and slowly winning over the brains and hearts of our best Germans, the lack of organization ensured that no racial hygiene measures could be taken. The importance of racial hygiene has only become known in Germany to all intelligent Germans through the political work of Adolf Hitler, and it was only through him that our more than thirtyyear-old dream has become a reality and racial hygiene principles have been translated into action.

This article is to give expression of our deep gratitude to our Führer before the whole world.

Today the road to racial hygiene is clear. However, we have just taken the first few small steps on it and there are many, many more steps to come until the major goal of racial hygiene is accomplished. Racial Hygiene is no fashionable thing, it must accompany a race at all times so it can always remain on top. To organise our People and our Race in the future in accordance with the views of racial hygiene, to provide people with the implements the spiritual and moral equipment which are needed for this fateful journey, is the duty of the German Society for Racial Hygiene together with other organisations which through the offices of the Reichsminister Dr. Frick have been newly organised along racial lines.

Rüdin once again...

In his career Rüdin has had no shortage of well earned honours, and just recently he received the Goethe-Medaille für Kunst und Wissenschaft (Goethe Medal for Art and Science) "In recognition of his achievements in the development of German racial hygiene". The Reichsminister of the Interior Dr Frick sent him the following telegram of congratulation: 'To the unceasing pioneer of racial hygiene and the meritorious protagonist of racial hygienic measures in the Third Reich, I send my sincerest congratulations on his 65th birthday. May you be able to continue your research for the benefit of mankind for a long time to come.' The Wiesbaden Congress of German Psychiatrists, Neurologists and Internists presented him with the Erb-Medaille.

Angesichts dieser Laufbahn hat es Rüdin nicht an wohlverdienten Ehrungen gefehlt, so erhielt er noch jüngst vom Führer die Goethe-Medaille für Kunst und Wissenschaft "In Anerkennung seiner Verdienste um die Entwicklung der deutschen Rassenhygiene". - Der Reichsminister des Innern Dr. Frick übersandte ihm das folgende Glückwunschtelegramm: "Dem unermüdlichen Vorkämpfer der Rassenhygiene und verdienstvollen Wegbereiter für die rassenhygienischen Maßnahmen des Dritten Reiches sende ich zum 65 Geburtstage meine herzlichsten Glückwünsche. Möge es ihnen noch recht lange vergönnt sein, Ihre Forschung zum Wohl der Menschheit weiterzuführen". - Die Wiesbadener Tagung der Deutschen Psychiater, Neurologen und Internisten verlieh ihm die Erb-Medaille.

The Führer thanks Rüdin.

Schriften aus dem Rassenpolitischen Amt der NSDAP
bei der Gauleitung Mainfranken zum Dr.-Hellmuth-Plan

Werner Schneider

Die Entmannungen
in Mainfranken in den Jahren
1934-1936

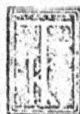

1937

Verlag Konrad Triltsch Würzburg-Aumühle

*One of the publications of the Racial-Political department of the
NSDAP, headed by Rüdin's colleague Dr. A. Gütt.*

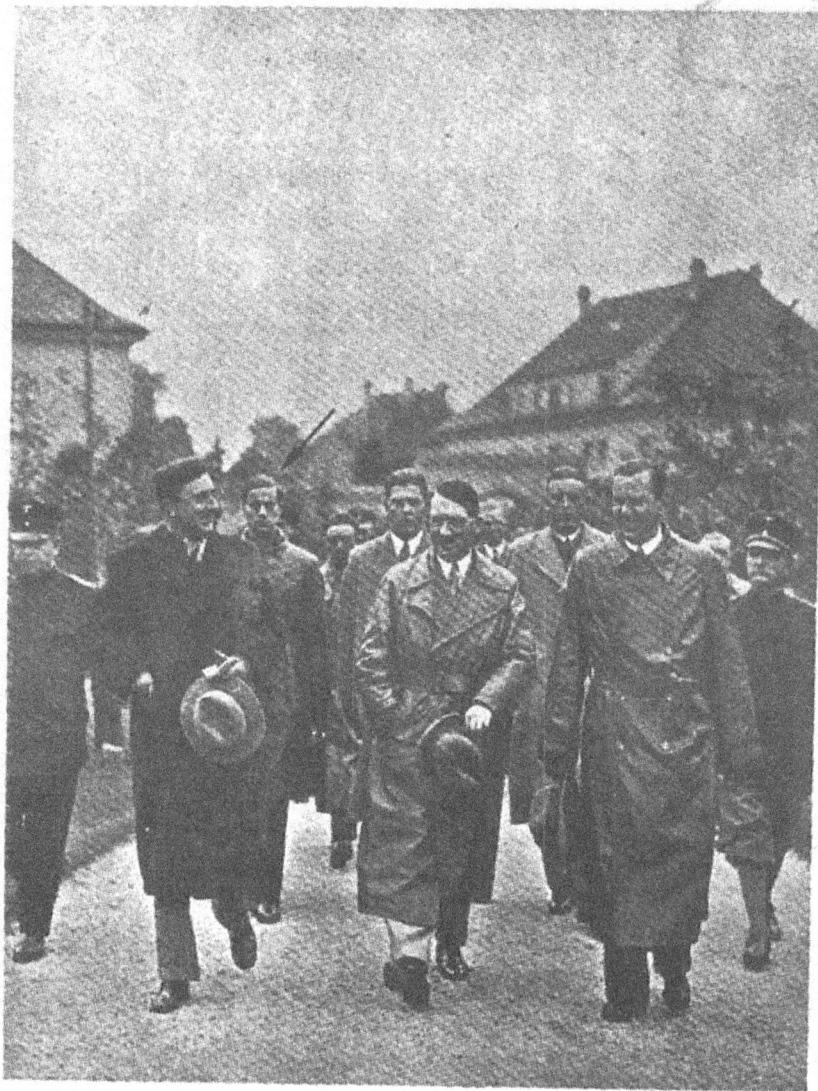

Hitler revisits his former prison. Behind him the grey eminence Dr. Karl Brandt.

Abgabe-Anstalt: *S c h u s s e n r i e d*   *durchgeführt am 9. Juli 1940*

Lfde. Nr.	Name und Vorname	T- Nr.	K- Nr.	Geburtsort und -tag	
1	Bürkle, Klara			Grötzingen	30. 12. 98
* 2	Fischer, Theresia			Röthardt	19 6. 00
3	Kahn, Jeanette, Sara			Gemmingen	18. 11. 70
4	Knoll, Maria geb. Wannenwetsch			Stuttgart	25. 7. 97
5	Knörnschild, Maria			Heidenheim	22. 3. 11
* 6	Koch, Helene			Heilbronn	12. 6. 63
7	Kögel, Ursula			Unterweiler	13. 9. 79
8	Kraus, Anna			Gaishardt	2. 3. 36
9	Kraut, Bertha			Schöntal	30. 6. 72
10	Kuch, Magdalene			Klopfhof	30. 9. 93
11	Kuhnle, Emilie			Unterbalzheim	9. 9. 93
12	Kurz, Karoline			Mittelstadt	28. 3. 95
* 13	Laidig, Elise			Steinheim	3. 4. 93
14	Lange, Anna			Rheinzabern	18. 6. 01
15	Lenzenhuber, Rosa			Obersulmetingen	6, 3. 99
16	Leute, Margarete geb. Bass			Heidenheim	17. 2. 95
17	Liebert, Klara geb. Wenig			Wildbad	7. 9. 98
* 18	Lindacher, Bertha			Elchingen	26. 9. 80
19	Löw, Lina			Heilbronn	8. 4. 89
* 20	Ludwig, Margarete geb. Maier			Schnaitheim	22. 7. 78
21	Maier, Theresia			Aepfingen	14. 7. 00
* 22	Mailänder, Elisabeth, geb. Maier			Nattheim	10. 10. 04
23	Martinelli, Theodosia			Reval	4. 9. 74
24	Mauch, Elisabeth			Rottenburg	19. 11. 76
* 25	Mayer, Katharine			Weiler	2. 6. 78
26	Meckle, Cäcilie geb. Weber			Dorfmerkingen	18. 11. 94
27	Meiser, Maria geb. Banzhaff			Heilbronn	4. 3. 95
* 28	Merk, Rosa geb. Eisele			Obereggatsweiler	16. 11. 65
29	Meyer, Dorothea geb. Reyhle			Göttingen	4. 5. 90
30	Müller, Creszentia geb. Wexel			Obergünzburg	22. 4. 84
31	Müller, Hilda			Ellwangen	2. 11. 11
32	Müller, Rosine			Ebersbach	24. 4. 94
33	Müller, Theresia			Saulgau	4. 7. 62
34	Müller, Viktoria			Reichenbach	5. 1. 86
35	Munding, Josefine geb. Bodon			Mühlhausen	16. 3. 84

This is what the transport lists of T4 looked like.

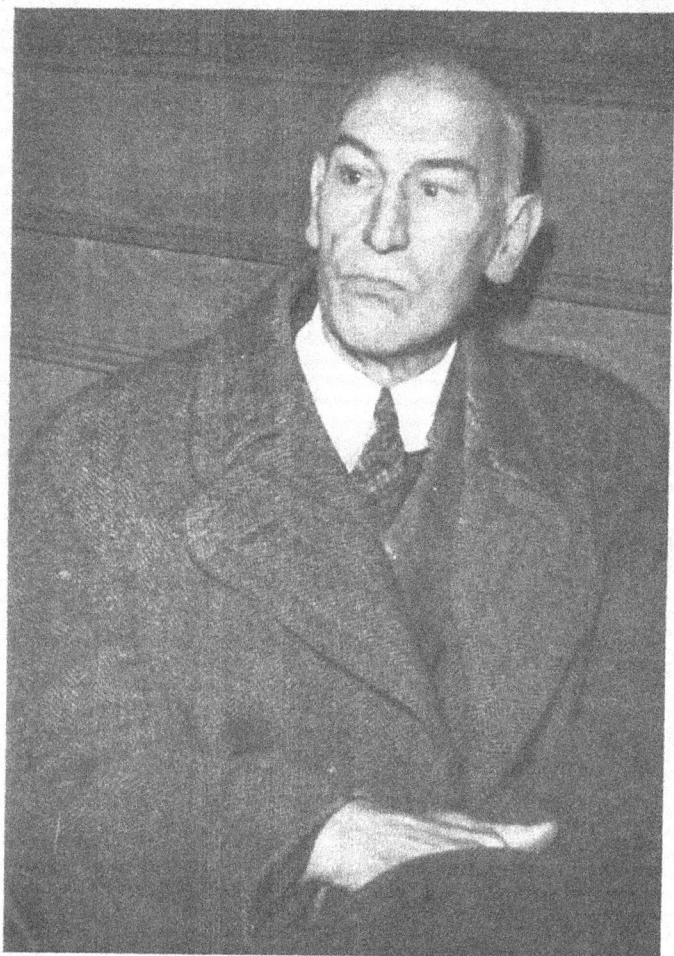

Dr. Adolf Wahlmann, Hadamar murder chief.

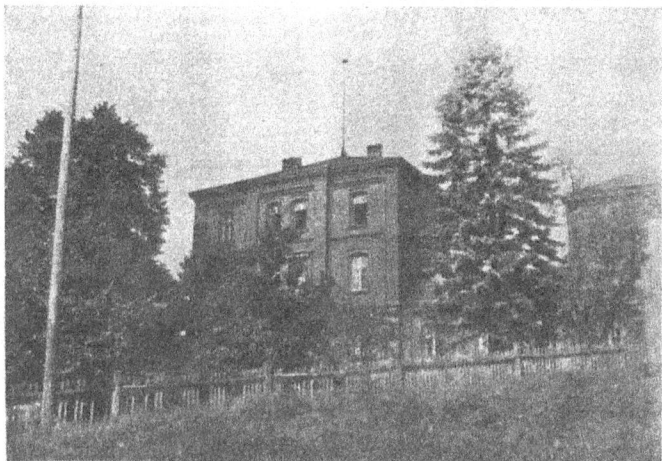

Front view of the Hadamar Institution. Quietly and peacefully...

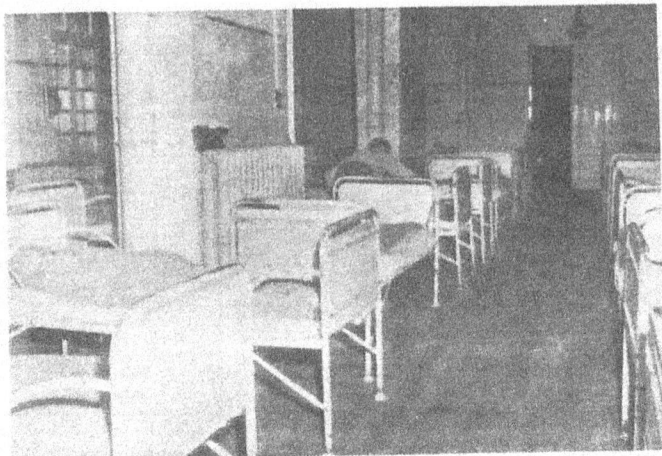

Ward 1B. Hadamar Institution. ...they died here.

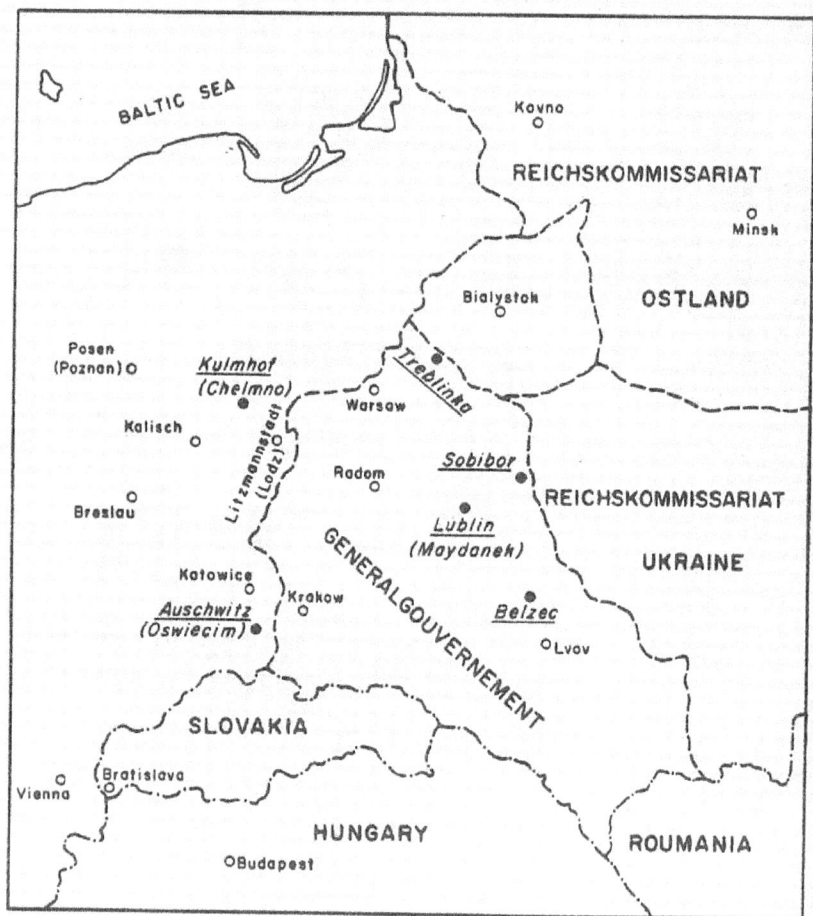

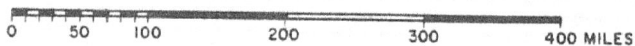

THE KILLING CENTERS

The Medical Machine of Destruction*

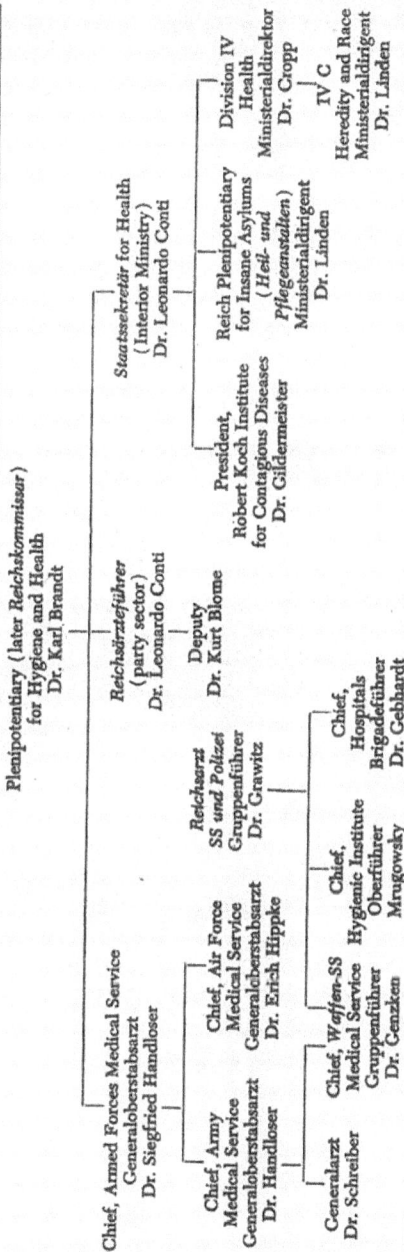

Plenipotentiary (later *Reichskommissar*) for Hygiene and Health
Dr. Karl Brandt

Chief, Armed Forces Medical Service
Generaloberstabsarzt
Dr. Siegfried Handloser

- Chief, Army Medical Service, Generaloberstabsarzt, Dr. Handloser
- Chief, Air Force Medical Service, Generaloberstabsarzt, Dr. Erich Hippke
- Generalarzt, Dr. Schreiber
- Chief, *Waffen-SS* Medical Service, Gruppenführer, Dr. Genzken
- Chief, Hygienic Institute, Oberführer, Mrugowsky

Reichsärzteführer (party sector)
Dr. Leonardo Conti

Deputy
Dr. Kurt Blome

- *Reichsarzt SS und Polizei*, Gruppenführer, Dr. Grawitz
  - Chief, Hospitals, Brigadeführer, Dr. Gebhardt

Staatssekretär for Health (Interior Ministry)
Dr. Leonardo Conti

- President, Robert Koch Institute for Contagious Diseases, Dr. Gildermeister
- Reich Plenipotentiary for Insane Asylums (*Heil- und Pflegeanstalten*), Ministerialdirigent, Dr. Linden
- Division IV Health, Ministerialdirektor, Dr. Cropp
  - IV C Heredity and Race, Ministerialdirigent, Dr. Linden

*Based upon: Chart, signed by Dr. Karl Brandt, undated, NO-845, and *Taschenbuch für Verwaltungsbeamte,* 1943, PS-3475.

Extermination Camp Treblinka. T4 plan of a death camp: The buildings are situated in an efficient manner.

Vergleichen Sie die Namensliste mit der Aufzählung der Namen der Eugenics Society 1932 – 1933.

...mpare this list of names with the list of names of the Eugenics Society of 1932-1933.

COMPOSITION OF GROUPS

The names of people who joined groups but did not attend their sessions regularly have been omitted from this list.

GROUP 1(A): **TECHNIQUES OF MENTAL HEALTH IN SCHOOLS FOR NORMAL CHILDREN.**

Chairman: Dr. A. F. Alford (*U.K.*); *Secretary*: Mr. R. Howlett (*U.K.*); *Belgium*: Mlle. M. Declercq, Mr. H. Dekegel, Mr. R. Deriviere, Mr. P. Gobert, Dr. A. M. Laporta, Mlle. S. Vandergucht; *Sweden*: Mrs. Gillqvist; *U.K.*: Dr. Mary Ferguson, Mr. A. J. Lilliman.

GROUP 1(B): **TECHNIQUES OF MENTAL HYGIENE IN SCHOOLS FOR ABNORMAL CHILDREN.**

Chairman: Dr. A. Friedemann (*Switzerland*); *Secretary*: Dr. T. A. Ratcliffe (*U.K.*); *Belgium*: Mlle. L. Dekeukelaire, Dr. A. Dourlet, Dr. H. Hoven, Mlle. C. Mutsaers; *Egypt*: Mrs. Z. Trampides; *Israel*: Dr. Elise Dagoni-Weinberg; *Italy*: Dr. T. Detre; *Sweden*: Dr. Torsten Ramer; *U.S.A.*: Dr. R. E. Troy.

GROUP 2: **PRACTICAL MEASURES FOR THE EDUCATION OF TEACHERS IN PRINCIPLES OF MENTAL HEALTH.**

Chairman: Prof. I. M. Laird (*Canada*); *Secretary*: Mlle. E. Moritz (*Belgium*); *U.S.A.*: Dr. Reichenberg-Hackett, Dr. Irving Salan.

GROUP 3: **EDUCATION OF PROFESSIONAL WORKERS IN MENTAL HEALTH.**

Chairman: Dr. E. Gobbi (*Switzerland*); *Secretary*: Mme. Z. Jurzynska (*Belgium*); *Austria*: Dr. Wilhelm Solms; *Belgium*: Dr. Marcel Alexander, Dr. C. Andersen, Mlle. M. Blariaux, Prof. E. De Craene, Mme. M. Detière, Mlle. Huynen, Mlle. A. Lempereur, Mlle. J. Stilmant, Mlle. G. Torchin, Mlle. E. Veekmans, Mlle. G. Willems; *Egypt*: Dr. S. Girgis, Dr. M. K. el Kholy; *Iraq*: Dr. M. K. Shabender; *Spain*: Dr. J. Pelach.

GROUP 4: **EDUCATION OF THE PUBLIC IN PRINCIPLES OF MENTAL HEALTH.**

Chairman: Dr. Doris Odlum (*U.K.*); *Secretary*: Miss M. Applebey (*U.K.*); *Austria*: Dr. Walter Spiel; *Belgium*: Mme. I. Becquart, Mme. O. Bodarwee, Dr. J. V. Z. Corbisier, Mlle. E. de Smedt, Mr. R. Vermeire; *Brazil*: Prof. A. C. Pacheco e Silva, Dr. A. Silveira; *Finland*: Miss E. K. Kajatsalo; *France*: Dr. Marcelle Geber, Mlle. Germaine Mercier; *Germany*: Prof. Dr. W. Villinger; *Portugal*: Dr. Baëta Neves; *South Africa*: Mrs. I. E. Gericke; *Sweden*: Miss I. Nyblaeus; *Switzerland*: Dr. Henri Bersot; *Turkey*: Prof. Kerim-Gökay; *U.K.*: Alderman W. J. Garnett; *U.S.A.*: Miss S. Maynard, Dr. B. H. Roberts, Mr. R. C. Roy; *Yugoslavia*: Mr. Leo Baric.

GROUP 5: **PROVISION AND MANAGEMENT OF DAY CENTRES (CRECHES) FOR CHILDREN OF PRE-SCHOOL AGE.**

Chairman: Dr. C. Koupernik (*France*); *Secretary*: Mlle. L. Van Keerberghen (*Belgium*); *Belgium*: Mlle. Dr. M. T. Callewaert, Mme. Crutzen de Velden, Dr. S. Deroy-Pasteel, Mlle. G. Revelard, Mlle. M. R. Smets, Mr. H. Uyttersprot, Mr. E. De Vlaminck, Mlle. G. Wielemans; *Finland*: Dr. M. L. Koski; *Netherlands*: Dr. M. Vromen.

GROUP 6: **THE SOCIAL CARE OF BACKWARD AND MENTALLY HANDICAPPED PERSONS.**

Chairman: Miss R. S. Addis (*U.K.*); *Secretary*: Dr. R. Fidler (*U.K.*); *Belgium*: Dr. A. Piérard, Prof. M. Staffe, Mlle. Steinmetzer, Mme. J. van den Wouwer; *Italy*: Prof. Dr. C. de Sanctis.

GROUP 7: **PRACTICAL MEASURES FOR DEALING WITH THE MENTAL HEALTH PROBLEMS OF REFUGEES.**

Chairman: Miss Betty Barton (*U.S.A.*); *Secretary*: Mlle. Germaine Marichal (*Belgium*); *Belgium*: Mme. C. Collard-Fassin; *Finland*: Dr. Reino Lagus; *Germany*: Dr. Annelore Schulte, Frau Emma Schulze; *Israel*: Dr. A. A. Weinberg; *U.S.A.*: Dr. T. F. Dwyer, Dr. Dallas Pratt, Dr. Norman Zinberg.

GROUP 8: **TECHNIQUES OF MENTAL HYGIENE IN THE INDUSTRIAL FIELD.**

Chairman: Dr. Leo H. Bartemeier (*U.S.A.*); *Germany*: Prof. Dr. K. Coerper; *Sweden*: Mr. E. Pihlgren, Mr. B. M. Gillqvist.

GROUP 9: **MENTAL HEALTH AND THE WORK OF THE NURSE.**

Chairman: Dr. W. Ironside (*U.K.*); *Secretary*: Dr. Mary Hemingway-Rees (*U.K.*); *Belgium*: Mme. J. Benoit, Mlle. Dr. Draps; *U.K.*: Dr. A. Milne, Miss A. Powell; *U.S.A.*: Capt. Esta Carini, Capt. Leota Moore.

Study groups for the WFMH - Villinger with his overseas allies

114

ASSOCIATES OF WFMH
1960-1961

ARGENTINA (6)
Dr. Mario Allaria
Dr. René Baron
Prof. Dr. E. E. Krapf
Sra. E. E. Krapf
*Mrs. A. D. Martin
Dra. Norma Tobar

AUSTRALIA (19)
Dr. Lesley H. Barnes
Dr. Donald F. Buckle
Dr. Beryl G. Cooley
Dr. Judith E. Dey
*Dr. W. Andrew Dibden
*Miss Margaret Evans
Dr. F. W. Graham
Mrs. Barbara Hasslip
Dr. F. A. S. Jensen
Dr. Robert Kiel
Dr. R. V. Lea
Dr. K. E. Le Page
Dr. B. A. Longfield
Mr. J. A. McCall
Dr. Ainslie Meares
Dr. Bruce H. Peterson
Dr. W. F. Salter
Dr. G. H. Springthorpe
Dr. Alan Stoller

AUSTRIA (2)
Prof. Dr. Hans Hoff
Dr. Hans Strotzka

BELGIUM (8)
Dr. Marcel Alexander
Mme. N. Arcangel-Stievenart
Dr. Marie-Th. Callewaert
Prof. Dr. Jacques de Busscher
M. le Chanoine Elie Gallez
Dr. Gommaire Van Looy
Dr. G. Varenne
Mlle. Rosette Woestyn

BRAZIL (2)
Prof. Dr. A. C. Pacheco e Silva
Dr. Mario Yahn

CANADA (45)
Dr. Douglas E. Alcorn
Miss Marie A. Aprile
Dr. Karl S. Bernhardt
Rev. Swithun Bowers
Miss Ruth M. Bray
Mrs. J. G. Cameron
Mr. Vladimir B. Cervin
Dr. Brock Chisholm
Mrs. Brock Chisholm
Dr. François Cloutier
Dr. Henri F. Ellenberger
Dr. Max Florence
Mr. Herbert O. Frind
Dr. J. D. M. Griffin
Dr. Robert O. Jones
Dr. Margery King
Dr. R. G. N. Laidlaw
Prof. I. M. Laird
Dr. Ernest R. Laycock
Prof. William Line
Mrs. S. Mackay-Smith
Father Noel Mailloux, O.P.
Dr. Edward L. Margetts
Dr. Anna Martire
Dr. D. G. McKerracher
Mrs. R. C. McNeil
Dr. A. E. Moll
Dr. Dayanand Naidoo
Dr. Evangelos Papathomopoulos
Prof. R. W. Payne
Dr. Moe J. Raff
Mrs. Walter H. Rice
Dr. C. E. Robinson
Miss Lillian R. Romkey
Dr. C. T. Rousell
Dr. W. C. M. Scott
Dr. Austin Sewell
Mrs. M. N. Sherman
Dr. R. Bruce Sloane
Dr. Graham C. Taylor
Dr. J. S. Tyhurst
Mrs. Vincent Voaden
Mrs. Nell West
Dr. J. R. Wilson
Dr. Eric D. Wittkower

CEYLON (2)
Dr. James S. P. Abeyawardena
Dr. W. Grillmayr

CHILE (1)
Prof. Dr. Carlos Nassar

CHINA (8)
Dr. Chu-chang Chen
*Miss Lorna M. Horwood
Mrs. Mei-chen Lin
Prof. Dr. Tsung-yi Lin
Dr. Peng-shou Liu
Dr. Hsien Rin
Dr. M. C. Tsuang
Dr. Eng-kung Yeh

COLOMBIA (2)
Dr. Carlos A. Gonzalez-Caceres
Prof. Dr. Carlos A. León

COSTA RICA (1)
Prof. Mariano L. Coronado

CYPRUS (1)
Dr. A. P. Mikellides

CZECHOSLOVAKIA (1)
Prof. Dr. Jaroslav Stuchlik

DENMARK (9)
Dr. Karl O. Christiansen
Mr. J. A. Larsen
Mr. Ove Lundbye
Dr. Gudmund Magnussen
Mr. E. H. Norung
Mr. Kurt Palsvig
Dr. Paul J. Reiter
Mr. B. Borup Svendsen
Dr. Jarl Wagner-Smith

FINLAND (4)
Miss E. K. Kajatsalo
Prof. Niilo Mäki
*Dr. O. W. von Nandelstadh
Mr. Edwin Törmälä

FRANCE (21)
Prof. Henri Baruk
Dr. P. F. Chanoit
M. J. J. Comas
Dr. René Diatkine
Dr. Pierre Doussinet
Dr. J. Favez-Boutonier
Dr. Marcelle Geber
M. André Isambert
Dr. Courbaire de Marcillat
Dr. Hubert Mignot
Dr. Hiroshi Nakajima
M. l'Abbé Lucien Oziol
M. Félix Padoa
Dr. Charles L. Pidoux
Dr. Yves Porc'her
Mme. Alice Rividi
M. Jean Sarbourg
Prof. Paul Sivadon
Dr. Claude Veil
Dr. Jean de Verbizier
Dr. M.Th. Zangerlin

GERMANY (38)
Prof. Dr. W. von Baeyer
Dr. H. J. Baltrusch
Dr. med. Manfred ind er Beeck
Dr. Alexander Boroffka
*Frau Gretel Derbolowsky
*Dr. A. Dührssen
Frau Dr. Martha Friedlander
*Studienrat Joachim Fritzen
Dr. Leo Gesslein
*Dr. Charlotte Giese
Dr. med. Wilhelm K. Hagen
Dr. med. H. J. Hartenstein
*Dr. Magda Kelber
Miss Mary A. Kelleher
Dr. Rudolf Klaus
Dr. Karl Klüwer
Miss Gerda Knoche
*Dr. Christiane Koenigs
Dr. Bruno Lewin

Dr. G. Maetze
Dr. Ernst Mansfeld
Dr. med. Ruth Mattheis
*Dr. L. Mayer-Kulenkampff
Dr. Hans Merguet
Dr. Luise Merguet
Dr. Curt Meyer
Dr. Annette Neumann
Dr. Helmut Paul
Dr. Harald Petri
Dr. med Gertrud Philipp
*Dr. Anna Ronge
Mrs. Ruth Rudert
*Frau Emma Schulze
*Mrs. Eva Seligmann
*Dr. med. Gertrud Soeken
Dr. Renato Staewen
Frau Berthel Stahl
*Prof. Dr. Werner Villinger

GREECE (3)
Dr. N. N. Dracoulides
Dr. George M. Jacobides
Dr. George Lyketsos

INDIA (7)
Dr. P. B. Buckshey
Dr. Edna Gault
Mr. K. P. Nayak
Prof. J. J. Panakal
Mr. S. A. Sarkar
Dr. Bhagwan P. Shah
Dr. Shanti Sheth

IRAN (5)
Dr. H. Davidian
Prof. Mohamed Guilani
Dr. Said Hekmat
Dr. Abdol-Hossein Mir-Sepassy
Dr. E. Tchehrazi

IRELAND (6)
Dr. Peter Dempsey
Dr. V. J. Dolphin
Father Celestine Rhatigan
Dr. B. Lyons Thornton
Rev. Brother Vincent Tobin

ISRAEL (2)
Dr. Giulio E. J. Muggia
Dr. A. A. Weinberg

ITALY (5)
Dr. Rita T. Forte
Prof. Angeleri Franco
Dr. G. Migliorino
Prof. Dr. Carlo de Sanctis
Signora de Sanctis

JAPAN (1)
Dr. Tatsuo Shoji

KOREA (3)
Dr. Suk-Whan Oh
Dr. Petrus Suckjin Yoo
Dr. Joo Yong Soh

KUWAIT (1)
*Dr. Mohamed Talaat Reda

LIBERIA (1)
Dr. Henrique Benson

MAURITIUS (1)
Dr. A. C. Raman

NETHERLANDS (19)
Dr. M. R. van Alphen de Veer
Dr. P. A. H. Baan
Mr. A. Th. M. Bakker
Dr. A. J. H. Bartels
Mr. J. E. v.d. Bergh van Dantzig
Dr. C. W. du Boeuf
Prof. Dr. F. J. J. Buytendijk
Dr. S. J. P. Dercksen
Mr. A. A. P. Ferket
Rev. H. L. Goudt
Miss W. van Lanschot
Dr. Eugenia C. Lekkerkerker
Dr. A. Poslavsky

Prof. Dr. H. C. Rümke
Mrs. H. C. Rümke
Dr. H. Ruygers
Mrs. Anna Vali
Dr. F. Vriesendorp
Mr. A. J. Welman

NEW ZEALAND (7)
Mrs. Eva Fischman
Dr. Wallace Ironside
Dr. David H. Livingstone
Dr. R. W. Medlicott
Dr. med. Olga W. Semon
Dr. G. M. Tothill
Mrs. Margaret Wildman

NORWAY (2)
Dr. Bard Brekke
*Mag. Cato Hambro

PAKISTAN (1)
Dr. Mohammad Rashid Chaudhry

PERU (3)
Dr. Baltazar Caravedo
Dr. Juan Gonzalez-Maertens
Dr. Carlos A. Seguin

PHILIPPINES (23)
Dr. Benigno Aldana
Dr. Estafania Aldaba-Lim
Capt. Rodolfo P. Andal
Mr. Otilio A. Arellano
Prof. Pascasio S. Banaria
Dr. Domingo C. Bascara
Mr. Alfonso Calalang
Dr. José M. Clarin
Dr. Florencio Z. Cruz
Dr. Manuel Escudero
Dr. José A. Fernandez
Prof. Dolores S. Francisco
Dr. Gumersindo García, Sr.
Dr. Cesarea Goduco-Aguilar
Dean Feliciano Jover Ledesma
Mr. Alvaro L. Martinez
Mrs. Geronima T. Pecson
Dr. Asuncion A. Perez
Prof. Waldo S. Perfecto
Dr. Jesus M. Tan
Dr. Filemon Tanchoco, Jr.
Atty. Vicente de Vera
Dr. Jaime C. Zaguire

POLAND (3)
Prof. Dr. K. Dabrowski
Dr. Tadeusz Gnat
Prof. Dr. Zygmunt Kuligowski

PORTUGAL (3)
Dr. Carlos Alvim-Costa
Dr. Francisco Alvim
Prof. Vítor H. M. Fontes

SARAWAK (1)
Dr. K. E. Schmidt

SPAIN (9)
Prof. Juan Bosch Marin
Dr. Justo Díaz Villasante
Dr. E. Grañen
Dr. J. R. de Otaola
Dr. Juan Obiols Vie
Dr. Joaquin Pelach
Dr. José R. Radó
Prof. Dr. Ramón Sarró
Dr. R. Vidal-Teixidor

SUDAN (2)
Dr. Taha Baasher
Dr. Tigani M. El Mahi

SWEDEN (8)
Mr. Bengt Eriksson
Dr. George M. Jacobson
Dr. A. V. Lagercrantz-Hallberg
Mrs. Phyllis McGill Lindo
Mr. Gösta M. Nordfors
Miss Ingeborg Nyblaeus
Dr. Kurt Törnquist
Miss Gerd Zetterström

115

SWITZERLAND (46)
Dr. Georges Abraham
Dr. Anne Audéoud-Naville
Prof. Gaetano Benedetti
Dr. Norbert Reno
Dr. J. Bergier
Mme. Hélène Billard
Mlle. Rosy Boehler
Dr. Edmond Chatelain
Mme. Liliane Clerc
M. Jean-Pierre Dobbert
Dr. Sylvia Dupuis
Dr. Charles Durand
Dr. A. Favre
Dr. Harry Feldmann
Dr. Antoine de Féraudy
Dr. O. L. Forel
Prof. A. Francheschetti
M. Emil Frei
Dr. A. Friedemann
Dr. Elio Gobbi
Dr. M. Gressot
Dr. Carl Haffter
Dr. R. Henny
Mme. Gertrude Herberts
Dt. med. F. Meerwein
Dr. med. M. Meierhofer
Dr. André Melley
Prof. Dr. Heinrich Meng
Dr. Paul Nef
Dr. jur. F. Nuscheler
Dr. D. Panagiotopoulos
Dr. Maria Pister
Dr. André Repond
Dr. Marcel Roch
Dr. Elizabeth Rotten
Mme. Nanik de Rougemont
Dr. Jean Sarkissoff
Mlle. Jeanne Sauthier
Mme. X. Petter de Schégloff
Dr. Kate Schuftan
Dr. med. Fred Singeisen
Mlle. Nina Sixtel
Dr. med. C. G. Tauber
Prof. Marc-Henri Thélin
Mme. Linda Tobler
Dr. R. Voluter de Loriol

THAILAND (2)
Dr. Subha Malakul
Dr. Praesop Ratanakorn

TURKEY (7)
Prof. Dr. Ihsan Sükrü Aksel
Dr. Nezahat Arkun
Mme. Sadiye Artunkal
Dr. Cihat Atasev
Dr. Kemal Elbirlik
Dr. Erdogan Noyan
Dr. med. Michel Sion

UNION OF SOUTH AFRICA (47)
*Dr. L. D. Adler
Dr. B. Crowhurst Archer
Dr. P. H. L. Barker
*Mr. Harold Bayne
*Mrs. Rose Bayne
Dr. S. Berman
*Dr. Allan V. Bird
Dr. Maurice Blair
Dr. R. W. S. Cheetham
Dr. M. Russel Clarke
*Dr. Harold Cooper
Dr. Max Feldman
Dr. E. Frankel
Dr. S. Friedman
Dr. R. Geerling
*Mrs. Elaine Gericke
Dr. L. S. Gillis
Dr. Morris Ginsburg
Mr. R. P. Gluckman
Dr. G. J. Goldberg
Dr. Margaret Grindley-Ferris
*Dr. L. M. Jacobs
Dr. S. Jacobson
Dr. C. L. B. Jeppe
Dr. W. G. Joffe
Dr. S. M. Katz
Dr. Max Klass
Dr. F. H. Kooy
Dr. A. McE. Lamont
Prof. R. E. Lighton
Miss I. I. Marwick
Dr. J. W. Scott Millar
*Dr. H. Moross
*Mrs. H. Moross
Dr. Marie S. Paterson

Dr. David Perk
Dr. A. S. Rakusin
*Dr. F. W. Rayner
Dr. F. Reinhold
*Mr. D. Ryan
Prof. C. H. Schmidt
Dr. C. Shufitz
Mr. A. H. Steels
Mrs. A. H. Steels
*Dr. H. Leonard Sussman
Mr. A. P. Tweeddale
Mr. Carl Weavind

UNITED ARAB REPUBLIC (Province of Egypt) (6)
Dr. Sabry Girgis
Mrs. Sabry Girgis
Dr. M. K. el Kholy
Miss Safia Ismail Magdi
Miss Fawzeya Aly Makhlouf
Dr. A. Wagdi

UNITED KINGDOM and Overseas Dependencies (241)
Miss Robina S. Addis
*Dr. James W. Affleck
Dr. R. H. Ahrensfeldt
*Miss Priscilla R. Alldridge
Dr. M. W. Annear
*Dr. P. L. Backus
*Mrs. P. L. Backus
*Mr. Sydney Balsh-Ward
*Dr. R. F. Barbour
*Mrs. K. M. D. Barker
*Dr. Erasmus D. Barlow
Prof. Sir Frederic Bartlett
Dr. Eva Bene
*Dr. Donald A. S. Blair
*Miss R. T. Bonar
*Dr. John Bowlby
Dr. Felix Brown
*Mrs. Violet Browne
Miss Kate W. Bruce
*Miss Margaret P. Buchanan
*Miss M. St. L. Burke
*Dr. Charles Burns
*Dr. William G. Burrows
Rt. Hon. R. A. Butler
Major T. L. Callender
*Miss L. V. Cameron
*Dr. Mary Capes
*Dr. C. O. Carter
Dr. L. C. F. Chevens
Dr. H. I. Clapham
Mr. John A. Clark
*Dr. G. S. Clouston
Mrs. G. Considine
*Miss D. L. Cornish
Dr. Isobel B. Craighead
*Dr. E. M. Creak
*Dr. R. W. Crocket
Dr. Timothy Crowley
Dr. Edwin Crundwell
*Mrs. Winifred M. Curzon
*Sir Allen Daley
*Mrs. V. J. Davidson
Mrs. Arna K. H. Davis
Rev. David Dick
*Dr. Henry V. Dicks
Mr. Meyer Domnitz
Mrs. A. W. Douglas
*Mr. John B. Drake
Mr. Michael Dunwell
Dr. Harry Edelston
*Miss Margaret Eden
*Mr. John A. F. Ennals
*Dr. Phyllis V. L. Epps
Mr. H. J. Esson
*Dr. Mary Ferguson
*Dr. Joan Fitzherbert
Dr. Fleischhacker
Dr. C. M. Fleming
Dr. Miriam Florentin
Dr. Michael Fordham
Mr. Harley D. Frank
*Dr. Hugh L. Freeman
Dr. Charles Friedman
Dr. A. R. Garner
*Alderman W. J. Garnett
*Mr. Leslie Geach
Dr. S. S. Gilder
Dr. S. W. Gillman
Mrs. Grace Gittins
Dr. Samson Goldin
*Mrs. Sybil Goldsmith
*Sir Stuart Goodwin
Dr. Mary G. Gorrie
*Miss Ann A. Graham

Dr. Brenda Grant
Rev. Dr. J. P. Grant
Dr. T. E. Grant
Dr. W. H. Gratrix
Mrs. Mary Grechner
*Mr. E. Grunfeld
Mrs. June Halville
*Miss L. M. Hamilton
*Miss Marian W. Hamilton
Mr. E. M. Harborow
Prof. G. R. Hargreaves
*Miss D. E. Harvie
Dr. Margaret Heller
*Mr. Ian Henderson
Miss Mary Hendry
Miss Irene Herzberg
*Dr. E. J. C. Hewitt
*Dr. C. Lamorna Hingston
Dr. E. Graham Howe
*Miss M. G. Howell
Dr. Colette Inebnit
*Miss Zoe Jarrett
Mrs. Dorothy Johnson
Mrs. Louisa A. Johnston
Dr. William Johnston
*Dr. Kathleen Jones
Dr. H. B. Kedward
*Miss Jessica King
Dr. C. C. Lack
*Dr. M. P. Leahy
*Miss Phyllis M. Legh
Prof. Sir Aubrey Lewis
*Dr. E. O. Lewis
Dr. Nancy Lewis
Dr. Jan T. Leyberg
*Dr. W. V. Livingston
*Mrs. G. M. Lloyd-Jones
Dr. Margaret Lowenfeld
Dr. R. J. Lumsden
*Mr. George A. Lyward
Bailie A. B. Mackay
Dr. Stephen MacKeith
*Dr. the Hon. Walter S. Maclay
Miss Janet Macleod
Dr. Donald M. Macmillan
Mr. J. Manson
Miss Margaret Martin
Dr. Anne H. McAllister
Dr. W. F. McAuley
*Miss M. S. T. McCash
*Mrs. F. E. McCloughry
Dr. Helena M. McKnight
Miss McQuade
Mr. Hugh McRae
Dr. James B. McWhinnie
Mrs. R. G. Medley
*Dr. Margaret Methven
*Prof. W. M. Millar
Dr. C. G. Milliman
*Miss Enid Mills
*Mrs. H. H. Minden
*Dr. Alfred Model
Dr. J. N. Morris
*Mr. F. D. Mott
*Mr. R. M. Mowbray
*Mrs. Lydia Mundy
*Miss D. A. Newlyn
Dr. Ralph A. Noble
*The Lady Norman
Mrs. D. L. O'Brien
Miss Nora L. Odell
*Dr. Doris M. Odlum
Dr. J. J. O'Reilly
Dr. Mangalore Narasimha Pai
*Mr. A. C. L. Paton
Dr. J. D. W. Pearce
Dr. G. R. Peberdy
*Mrs. Edna M. Phillips
*Dr. William Phillips
Dr. Francis Pilkington
Dr. T. L. Pilkington
*Dr. Mildred Pott
*Dr. T. A. Ratcliffe
Miss C. M. Rees
Miss Helen E. Rees
*Dr. J. R. Rees
*Mr. R. T. Rees
Dr. T. P. Rees
*Dr. Benjamin Reid
Miss C. A. Renton
Dr. Derek Richter
Mr. James Robb
*Mrs. M. E. Robert
Mr. James Robertson
*Dr. W. M. Ford Robertson
*Prof. T. Ferguson Rodger
Miss Margaret Rowlands
Dr. P. K. Roy
*Dr. Gerald de M. Rudolf

Dr. W. Schindler
*Dr. Harry Selby
Dr. F. Tindale Shadforth
Dr. David Shaw
*Dr. Elisabeth Shoenberg
*Dr. Myre Sim
*Miss Mary D. Smart
Miss Mabel F. Smith
*Dr. Kenneth Soddy
*Mrs. Kenneth Soddy
*Dr. Erwin Stengel
*Dr. Jeannie E. Stirrat
*Dr. F. H. Stone
Mrs. Helen C. Sutherland
*Dr. J. D. Sutherland
Mrs. N. Tarlton
*Dr. G. Teruel
Dr. D. H. H. Thomas
*Dr. A. S. Thorley
*Mr. E. A. Thornton
*Miss E. M. Thornton
Miss Jenifer Thuell
*Miss B. E. Towler
*Dr. Roger F. Tredgold
Sir Geoffrey Vickers
*The Lady Wakehurst
Miss Ada Waldy
Miss Dorothy M. Waldy
Mrs. C. H. Webb
Dr. Alastair J. Weir
*Mrs. Mary Welch
Miss Gladys A. Wheelband
Miss E. G. White
Mr. Daniel Whitelaw
Miss K. M. Whittington
*Dr. John F. Wilde
*Dr. Arthur H. Williams
*Dr. Isabel G. H. Wilson
*Miss Eileen L. Younghusband

Barbados
Dr. R. M. Lloyd Still

Hong Kong
Dr. Stephen Chang
Miss K. Y. Chen
Dr. Irene Cheng
Dr. Gerald Choa
Prof. Daphne Chun
Dr. Chung Chung Ho
Miss Daphne Ho
Mrs. Yue Heng Ho-Kan
Mrs. Eric Hotung
Miss Tsui-Ping Huang
Mrs. V. J. Jasper
Mrs. Anita K. Li
Dr. K. D. Ling
Miss Yi Ying Ma
Dr. the Hon. D. J. M. Macke
Miss Madge Newcombe
Prof. K. E. Priestley
Miss J. E. Rowe
Rev. L. Stumpf
Dr. the Hon. P. H. Teng
Dr. Pow Meng Yap
Dr. K. C. Yeo

Jamaica
*Dr. H. Feldman

Kenya
Miss I. M. Farmer

Singapore
*Miss Rita McEwan

Southern Rhodesia
Mr. H. H. Hall

Tanganyika
Dr. Cyril Smartt

Trinidad
Mrs. Nesta Patrick

UNITED STATES and its Territories (1427)
Dr. Theodora M. Abel
Miss Evelyn Abelson
*Dr. Joseph Abrahams
Dr. Teodora Abramovitch
Mr. Alvin Abrams
Dr. D. W. Abse
*Mr. Robert H. Ackerman
*Mrs. Robert H. Ackerman
Dr. Robert S. Adams
Mrs. Beatric G. Adkins
*Mrs. Evelyn D. Adlerblum
*Mr. Arthur Adlerstein
Mrs. Nancy L. Adsett
Dr. Alcinda P. de Aguiar
Dr. Mehmet S. Akaydin

116

117

Dr. Kenneth Gaver
Dr. David Geddes
Dr. Sara G. Geiger
*Dr. F. V. Geiss
Mr. Paul-Marcel Gelinas
Dr. Joseph J. Geller
Dr. Edward Gendel
Dr. Otto L. Gericke
Dr. Louis H. Gerstay
*Miss Ruth Gilbert
*Miss Eleanore Gill
Mrs. Louis S. Gimbel, Jr.
Mrs. Esther Goetz Gillialand
Mrs. Ethel L. Ginsburg
Dr. Maxwell Gitelson
*Miss Rebecca Glasmann
Dr. Alan James Glasser
Dr. Erik Glud
Dr. Eleanor T. Glueck
Prof. Sheldon Glueck
*Mrs. Louis Goldburt
Dr. Sidney S. Goldensohn
Miss Rose Goldman
Mr. Charles S. Goldsmith
Mrs. Charles S. Goldsmith
Dr. Jewett Goldsmith
Mrs. Carl Goldstein
Dr. Joseph L. Goldstein
Miss Mary A. Goodman
Dr. Richard E. Gordon
*Dr. Soll Goodman
Mr. John V. Gorton
Dr. Anna J. Gosline
*Mrs. Raymond Gosslin
Dr. Leon Gottfried
Mr. William J. Gough
*Miss G. M. Graham
Mrs. Helen Gravess
*Miss Winifred S. Graves
*Dr. Donald C. Greaves
*Dr. Maurice R. Green
*Mrs. J. Greene
*Dr. Marjorie Greene
Mrs. Robert F. Greene
Dr. Ralph R. Greenson
*Dr. Edward D. Greenwood
Miss Mary Greer
*Mrs. Henry Gregor
*Dr. Ian Gregory
*Mr. Robert Hays Gries
*Mrs. Robert Hays Gries
Dr. D. Park Griffin
Dr. W. R. Griswold
*Miss Ruth Groves
Mrs. Sidonie Gruenberg
Dr. Max Gruenthal
Mrs. Nahman H. Grunberg
*Mrs. Randolph Guggenheimer
Mrs. R. Joan Guilmartin
Mr. Ralph B. Guinness
Capt. Olga Gull
Dr. Meyer A. Gunther
Mr. John C. Gustin
Dr. Oskar Guttmann
Mrs. Vivian S. Guze
Mrs. Nora Hackel
Dr. Frederick J. Hacker
Dr. Samuel B. Hadden
Mrs. Florence Hagee
*Mrs. Ernestine R. Haight
Miss Madeleine Half
*Miss Jane Hall
*Miss Monica M. Haller
Mrs. June Halpern
Miss Sylvia Halpern
Mrs. Anita Halpert
Dr. Henry N. Hamilton
Dr. Ernet Hamburger
*Mrs. Jerome J. Hanauer
Mr. Norman Handelman
Miss Virginia R. Hannon
*Dr. Eldred F. Hardtke
*Mrs. Albert Haring
Mr. Albert J. Harris
*Mrs. Arthur K. Harris
Dr. Cecil Harris
Dr. Herbert I. Harris
Dr. June Harris
Dr. Titus H. Harris
Dr. Molly R. Harrower
Dr. Dora Hartmann
Dr. Edward O. Hascall, Jr.
Dr. Cosa Dell Haskell
Prof. Starke R. Hathaway
*Dr. Elsie L. Haug
Dr. George O. Haydu
*Mrs. Douglas Hays
Dr. Raymond Headlee
Dr. Lionel M. Heiden

Mrs. Vincent Heig
*Mr. Bernard Heineman
*Mr. Henry E. Heiner
*Mrs. Henry E. Heiner
Dr. Florence Heisler
Di. A. A. Hellams
*Mr. William B. Heller
*Mrs. William B. Heller
Dr. Helen C. K. Hendin
Dr. Edwin Henry
Mrs. Edythe M. Herson
Mr. Leo Herson
Mr. Richard J. L. Herson
*Miss Lucile M. Higby
Rev. Kenneth Hildebrand
Mrs. H. N. Hill
*Dr. Leonard E. Himler
*Mrs. Marcus Hirsch
*Dr. Ada Hirsh
*Mrs. L. A. Hockstader
*Mr. Fred K. Hoehler
Mr. Joe R. Hosler
*Mrs. Joseph F. Hoffman
Dr. Louis Hoffman
Dr. R. Holzer
*Miss Marguerite Holmes
Dr. Alvin Honigsberg
Dr. Prynce Hopkins
*Miss Edith M. Horstman
Miss Geraldine B. Howard
Mr. Stuart P. Howell
*Mr. Sherman R. Hoyt
*Mrs. Sherman R. Hoyt
Miss Mary A. Hulbert
Dr. Wilfred C. Hulse
Dr. Leopold A. Humar
*Miss Rosetta Hurwitz
Miss Biete Huseth
Mrs. Erika R. Hyde
Mrs. Martha Hynning
*Mr. D. John Heyman
Dr. Felix M. Ibanez
Miss Dolores Iltis
*Mrs. Donald Iseman
*Mrs. Henry Littlesdn
Dr. Evelyn P. Ivey
*Dr. Edith U. Jackson
*Miss Harriet A. Jackson
Dr. Seymour B. Jacobson
Mr. Herbert Jaffey
*Mr. Hubert E. James
Miss Victoria E. James
*Mrs. Margarethe Jauch
Dr. Benjamin Jeffries
Mrs. Kay Wade Jenkins
Dr. Paul H. Jenkins
Dr. Lucie Jessner
*Dr. Clara Johns
Mrs. W. E. Johns
Dr. Paul E. Johnson
Miss Ruth F. Johnson
Mrs. V. H. Johnson
Dr. Roletta Jolly-Fritz
Mr. J. Barclay Jones
Dr. David M. Jordan
Dr. Leopold Jordan
Dr. Elizabeth M. Junken
*Mr. Adolph J. Kaback
*Dr. Goldie R. Kaback
Miss Audrey M. Kachelski
*Mrs. Asya L. Kadis
Dr. Ralph J. Kabana
Dr. David F. Kahn
Dr. Lothar B. Kalinowsky
Dr. Alfred Kamm
*Dr. Alex H. Kaplan
*Mr. J. M. Kaplan
*Mrs. J. M. Kaplan
Mrs. Katherine F. Kaplan
Dr. Michael Kaplan
Mrs. Edna Karlsruher
Dr. Etta Karp
*Mr. Robert N. Kastor
Mrs. Giska T. Kates
Mr. Michael E. Kates
*Dr. Cecilia G. Katz
Dr. Freda S. Kaufman
Mr. R. P. Kelisky
Mrs. R. P. Kelisky
Dr. Elizabeth Kelley
Miss Roberta M. Kellogg
*Dr. Harold Kelman
Mr. Morris Kelnicker
*Mr. Allan H. Kempner
*Mrs. Allan H. Kempner
*Miss Anna Kempshall
Dr. Marian Kenworthy
Miss Helen Kern
Dr. Howard M. Kern, Jr.

Miss Ethel Keshner
Dr. Judith S. Kestenberg
Mr. Daniel King
Dr. Joseph P. King
*Miss Carolyn B. Kinney
Dr. Rosemarie S. Kircher
Miss Mina Kirzofsky
Mrs. Maxine Kissam
Prof. David B. Klein
Dr. Emanuel Klein
*Dr. Harry Klein
Dr. Ralph Klein
Dr. Robert Kleiner
Mr. Bruno Klopfer
Dr. Robert P. Knight
*Mrs. Ruth M. Knight
Mr. Hugh Knowlton
*Mrs. Harry Knox
*Dr. Genevieve Knupfer
Mrs. Henry V. Kobin
Dr. G. Frances Koenig
Dr. Delbert M. Kole
Prof. Richard Kolm
Mr. Myron Koltay
Dr. George Kontaxopoulos
Mrs. Richard K. Korn
Miss Maurine Kornfeld
Miss Anne Korshakovska
Dr. Gregorio Kort
Dr. Haydee C. Kort
Dr. Frederic P. Kosbab
*Dr. Marianne E. Kosbab
*Mrs. Stephen A. Koshland
*Dr. Edward A. Kowalyk
Mr. Charles E. S. Kraemer
*Dr. Samuel H. Kraines
*Dr. Judith E. Kranes
Dr. Herbert D. G. Krieger
Major Elsie Krchnavi
Dr. Othilda Krug
*Mrs. Hoch Kubie
*Dr. Lawrence S. Kubie
*Mrs. Samuel L. Kuhn
Dr. Anna M. Kulka
Mrs. Maty S. Kunst
Miss Levine H. Kunz
Mr. Kurt Kurdi
Mrs. Diana Kurzband
Mrs. Harriet R. Kutik
Dr. Frank M. Lachmann
*Mr. Mortimer Lahm
Miss Denise La Hullier
Mr. Hal Lainson
Mr. John Lainson
Miss Therese Latancette
Dr. John P. Lambert
Mr. Corliss Lamont
Dr. David Landau
Dr. Felicia L. Landau
Miss Gertrude Landau
Dr. Louis Landman
Miss Agnes T. Landis
Dr. Helena P. Langer
*Dr. Charles L. Langsam
Mrs. Sam Langsdorf
Dr. H. C. Lansdell
*Dr. Helen Lanting
Mr. George H. Laporte
*Mr. Mary W. Lasker
*Miss Ruth Lassoff
Dr. Maurice W. Laufer
*Miss Emma M. Layman
*Dr. Mary H. Layman
*Mrs. Fred Lazarus, Jr.
Miss Genevieve Lebendiger
*Dr. Lee Salk
Dr. Leon Lefer
*Hon. Herbert H. Lehman
Miss Melba Leichsenring
Dr. Alexander H. Leighton
Dr. Dorothy C. Leighton
Dr. Dorothea C. Leighton
Mr. J. M. Leitner
Dr. Henry L. Lennard
Mr. Theodore F. Lentz
Dr. A. S. Lentner
*Prof. Dr. Harold Leopold
Dr. Harry H. Lerner
*Mrs. Syril Lerner
Dr. Stanley Lesse
*Mrs. Marjorie F. Lesser
Dr. David Lester
Mrs. F. P. Lester
Miss Katharine E. LeVan
*Dr. Edgar A. Levenson
*Mrs. Robert H. Levi
Miss Leah Levinger
*Mrs. George E. Levinrew
*Dr. David M. Levy

*Dr. Norman J. Levy
Dr. Robert Levy
*Miss Garland K. Lewis
Dr. Murray D. Lewin
*Dr. Ray Lewis
Miss Ruth L. Lewis
*Dr. Marjorie Lewisohn
*Mr. Herman N. Liberman
Dr. Daniel Liebermann
Mrs. J. Lieberman
Dr. Samuel Liebman
*Dr. Harold I. Lief
*Dr. Pim W. K. Ligthart
Mrs. Charles H. Lillienfeld
Dr. Edward A. Lincoln
Dr. Walter Lingens
*Dr. Louis Linn
Dr. Theodore Lipin
Mrs. Martin Lippman
Dr. Daniel M. Lipshutz
Dr. Harry R. Lipton
Dr. Don C. Littlefield
Prof. Robert Livingston
*Mr. Carl M. Loeb
*Mrs. Carl M. Loeb
Mrs. Harry W. Loeb
*Mr. Henry Loeb
*Mrs. Henry Loeb
*Mrs. John L. Loeb
Mrs. Martin B. Loeb
Mrs. Eleanor Adams Loija
Dr. Jack B. Lomas
*Mr. Sandor Lorand
*Mrs. Sandor Lorand
Mr. Irving Lorge
Miss Dorine Loso
Dr. George M. Lott
Mr. Bolton Love
*Mrs. Madeleine M. Low
*Mr. David L. Luke, Jr.
*Mr. Sven Lundstedt
Mr. Leon M. Lurie
Mr. Edward E. Lustbader
*Mr. J. Lyle
*Dr. Curt L. Lynn
*Miss Elizabeth Lyon
Mr. James S. Lyons
*Mrs. Samuel MacElfatrick
Mr. James L. MacKay
Dr. Bett MacLeech
Miss Terry Macleod
Dr. Anna Maenchen
Dr. Philip M. Margolis
*Mr. James L. Magrish
Dr. Leonard T. Maholick
Mr. James S. Mahon
Mr. George Mally
Miss Edna Mann
Miss Elizabeth Mann
Mrs. Henry March
Dr. Allen S. Mariner
*Dr. Oskar B. Markey
Dr. Jacob L. Marks
Dr. Alfred J. Marrow
Dr. Elias J. Marsh
*Dr. Alexander Reid Martin
Miss Ruth M. Martin
*Dr. Johann R. Marx
*Mr. Leonard Marx
*Mrs. Leonard Marx
*Dr. Jules H. Masserman
*Mr. Erard A. Matthiessen
Miss Ella Mattson
*Mr. Baldwin Maull
*Mrs. Baldwin Maull
*Mr. Clinton O. Mayer, Jr.
*Mr. Frank D. Mayer
*Mrs. Jane Mayer
*Mrs. Paul Mazur
Mr. Marvin Marza
Mrs. Mary T. McAuliffe
Prof. Elizabeth McBroom
*Mrs. Ruth O. McCarn
*Dr. James L. McCartney
Dr. Sam G. McClellan
*Dr. Robert J. McCracken
Dr. William E. McCullou
Miss Roslyn G. McDona
Miss Elizabeth D. McDo
*Dr. Rosa A. McFarland
Dr. Alan A. McLean
Dr. Helen V. McLean
Miss Romayne McMaho
Mrs. R. C. McNeil
Dr. Margaret Mead
Mr. Charles R. Meeker
Mrs. Goldie Meenes
Professor Max Meenes
*Mr. Pebody C. Mehun

119

Miss Ellen Steinberg
*Dr. Louis D. Steinberg
*Dr. Meta H. Steiner
Mrs. Alexander Steinert
Mrs. Florence S. Stellern
Dr. M. G. Stemmermann
Mrs. Harriet Sterling
Dr. Harry Sterling
Mrs. W. M. Sterling
*Mrs. B. Albert Stern
*Miss Faith Stern
Mr. George A. Stern
*Mrs. George A. Stern
*Mrs. Herbert L. Stern
Mr. Leo C. Stern
Dr. Mark E. Stern
Dr. Morton M. Stern
*Mr. Rupert Stern
Dr. George S. Stevenson
Miss Florence H. Stewart
Dr. Paul R. Stimson
*Mrs. Ernest W. Stix
*Dr. Leo Stone
Prof. Helen F. Storen
*Mr. Pierre Straler
*Mrs. Pierre Straler
Dr. Frank B. Strange
*Mrs. Edna W. Strasser
*Mr. Frederick W. Straus
Miss Isabella R. Straus
Dr. Hans Strauss
*Mrs. Leonard Strauss
*Mrs. Julian Street
*Mrs. Florence B. Stroll
Miss G. E. L. Stromwall
Mr. Alan M. Stroock
Dr. J. N. P. Struthers
*Mrs. W. K. Sturges
Dr. Carl Sugar
Dr. Charles W. Sult
Miss Marion Sutherland
Dr. Keith Sward
Dr. Jacob Swartz
Dr. Harvey Sweetbaum
*Mrs. A. Lloyd Symington
Dr. Firooz N. Tabrizi
Dr. Luigi Tagliacozzo
Dr. Frank F. Tallman
Dr. Sidney L. Tamarin
Dr. Gerald Tannenbaum
Dr. Sidney Tarachow
*Dr. Hertha Tarrasch
Dr. Helen H. Tartakoff
Dr. Fred U. Tate
Dr. Hugo Taussig
Dr. Donald Taylor
*Miss Katharine Taylor
Dr. Katharine W. Taylor
Dr. Victor J. Teichner
Miss Hazel Teitzel
*Dr. William Terhune

Mr. Edward Terner
Dr. Ross Thalheimer
*Dr. Theodore Thass-Thienemann
Dr. Elizabeth Thoma
Dr. Alexander Thomas
Dr. Ruth H. Thomson
Dr. Charles B. Thompson
*Mrs. Charles G. Thompson
Prof. Clare Wright Thompson
*Dr. Lloyd J. Thompson
Mr. Robert Thorn
Mrs. Sonya F. Thorp
*Dr. Nelly Tibout
Dr. Charles W. Tidd
*Mrs. G. D. Tillinghast
Dr. Lawrence Tirnauer
Mrs. M. E. Tirrell
Mr. Leonard Titelman
Mrs. Leonard Titelman
Miss Helen M. Towey
Miss Yaye Togasaki
Mr. Louis J. Torre
Dr. Mottram Torre
*Mrs. Elisabeth M. Toth
*Mrs. Ronald Tree
Mrs. Phyllis F. Treusch
Dr. M. A. Tarumianz
Miss Millicent M. Tschaepe
Mrs. Annie L. Tucker
*Mrs. Milton H. Tucker
Dr. Alan B. Tulipan
*Mr. Ira H. Tulipan
Dr. Petras Tunkunas
Dr. Rodolph H. Turcotte
Dr. Louis L. Tureen
Dr. Robert Turfboer
Dr. Ann Ruth L. Turkel
Dr. Elizabeth F. Turnauer
Dr. Doris Twitchell-Allan
Miss Mirian Ungar
Dr. Arnold H. Ungerman
Mrs. Bess Z. Ungerman
Dr. Milford S. Ungerman
Mrs. Augusta Rubin Ury
Mr. A. L. Van Ameringen
*Dr. Bella S. Van Bark
Mrs. Genee E. VanSant
*Mrs. Gertrude Veit
Mr. C. Frank Velkas
Prof. Dr. George Vlavianos
Dr. Maria R. Vlavianos
Miss B. D. Wade
Mr. Nathaniel N. Wagner
Mr. Samuel Waldfogel
Dr. Marguerite Walker
Miss Mary Walker
Miss Clara Walter
Mrs. Margaret Walters
Dr. James D. Wang
Miss Claudia Wannamaker

Mr. Paul W. Wanner
*Dr. Bettina Warburg
Dr. M. La Vinia Warner
Dr. Geraldine Fink Wasserman
Dr. Morris Wasserman
Mrs. Roslyn Watman
Mr. Albert G. Watson
*Dr. Andrew S. Watson
Dr. Gladys H. Watson
Dr. George J. Wayne
*Prof. Dr. David Wdowinsky
*Dr. William F. Weber
*Dr. Bryant M. Wedge
Dr. Edith Weigert
Miss Blanche C. Weill
*Mr. Paul K. Weinandy
Miss Hannah Brodie Weiner
Dr. Paul S. Weiner
Mrs. Jane Weinrich
*Dr. William Weisdorf
Mrs. Frances Weiss
*Dr. Frederick A. Weiss
*Mrs. Julian D. Weiss
*Mrs. Louis S. Weiss
Miss M. Olga Weiss
Mrs. Myrna Weissman
*Mrs. Marion S. Wells
Miss Marianne Welter
Miss Katharine Abbot Wells
Mrs. Hans Wendel
*Mr. Gerald Wendt
Dr. Simon I. Wenkart
Mrs. L. Werbner
*Miss Marcella Werra
*Mr. Harris K. Weston
*Mrs. Harris K. Weston
Dr. Simon Weyl
Miss Lilyan T. Weymouth
*Mr. Morgan D. Wheelock
*Mrs. Morgan D. Wheelock
Miss Helen M. Whitbeck
Dr. Joseph B. Wheelwright
Mr. Joseph B. Wheelwright
Mr. Gilbert F. White
Mrs. Veleda White Sickels
*Mrs. Clarence Whitehill
Dr. John D. Whitehouse
Dr. Winifred G. Whitman
Dr. Benjamin Wiesel
Mrs. E. L. Wilbur
Dr. Katherine W. Wilcox
*Dr. Paul H. Wilcox
Dr. Paul G. Williams
*Miss Ruth M. Williams
Rev. Russell S. Williams
Dr. Stanley Willis
*Mr. Thomas E. Wilson
Dr. Herbert Winston
*Mr. Nathaniel Winthrop
*Mrs. Nathaniel Winthrop
Dr. Robert D. Wirt

*Dr. Florence Clothier Wis
Dr. John Harrison Wolave
*Colonel Arthur M. Wolf
Dr. S. Jean Wolf
Mr. William S. Wolf
Mrs. William S. Wolf
Dr. Ernst Wolff
Miss Margaret H. Wolff
*Mr. Alvin R. Wolfson
Miss Beatrice M. Wolfson
Dr. Rose Wolfson
*Mrs. M. Marian Wood
*Mrs. Julian L. Woodward
Mrs. D. H. Woodyard
*Dr. John J. Wooster
Miss Mary Elizabeth Wrig
Major Hanora Wright
*Dr. J. Allen Yager
Mr. C. H. Yalem
Mrs. Carrie Allen Young
Mr. Douglas Young
Miss Kay C. Young
Miss Myra S. Young
Mr. Gerald S. Yudkin
Dr. Lucy Zabarenko
Mrs. Vivian Zachary
Dr. Barbara Zambrowski
*Dr. Manuel D. Zane
Dr. George Zavitzianos
*Mrs. Blanche Zebine
Mr. Richard S. Zeisler
Dr. Valentine Wolf Zetlin
Dr. Isadore S. Zfass
Mrs. Isadore S. Zfass
Mrs. Samuel Zfass
Dr. I. Ziferstein
Mrs. Alice B. Zimmerman
*Miss Evelyn Zimmerman
*Dr. Kent A. Zimmerman
Dr. Norman Zinberg
*Mrs. Richard W. Zirinsky
*Dr. Eugene Ziskind
*Dr. Joseph M. Zucker

Hawaii
*Dr. Yan Tim Wong

Puerto Rico
Dr. Luis M. Morales

Virgin Islands
Mrs. Eldra L. M. Shulterbr

URUGUAY (1)
Dr. J. C. Chans Caviglia

VENEZUELA (3)
Dr. Carlos Gil Rincón
Dr. E. H. Ibanez Petersen
Dr. Fernando Valarino

YUGOSLAVIA (1)
Dr. Marty Gracina

NOTE.—An asterisk (*) indicates that more than the minimum annual subscription has been paid.

Professor Villinger and his fellow conspirators.

120

Officers and Executive Board 1968
Bureau et Conseil Exécutif 1968

*rofessor Dr. Ehrhardt, Villinger's protege has learned well and
arns his reward.*

Past Presidents of the Federation
Anciens Présidents de la Fédération

JOHN R. REES, M.D. (1948-1949)
Honorary President W.F.M.H., Formerly Director and Special Consultant World Federation for Mental Health London

DR. ANDRÉ REPOND (1949-1950)
Ancien directeur, Maison de santé de Malévoz, Monthey, Valais, Suisse

WILLIAM LINE, PH.D. † (1950-1951)
Professor of Psychology, Toronto

DR. ALFONSO MILLAN (1951-1952)
Professeur de psychiatrie, Mexico

M.K. EL KHOLY, M.D. (1952-1953)
Former Director-General, Department of Mental Diseases, Cairo

PROF. H.C. RÜMKE † (1953-1954)
Professor of Psychiatry, Utrecht, Netherlands

FRANK FREMONT-SMITH, M.D. (1954-1955)
Director, Interdisciplinary Conference Program, American Institute of Biological Sciences, New York

NIILO MAKI, PH.D. (1955-1956)
Professor of Special Education, Helsinki

PROF. E. EDUARDO KRAPF † (1956)
Chief, Mental Health Section, World Health Organization, Genève

MARGARET MEAD, PH.D. (1956-1957)
Associate Curator of Ethnology, American Museum of Natural History, New York

BROCK CHISHOLM, M.D. (1957-1958)
Victoria, British Columbia, Canada. Former Director-General, World Health Organization, Genève

PROF. HANS HOFF (1958-1959)
Professor of Neurology and Psychiatry, Vienna

PROF. PAUL SIVADON (1959-1960)
Professeur de psychiatrie et de psychologie, Bruxelles, directeur des Services de psychiatrie, Mutuelle Générale de l'Education Nationale, France

PROF. A.C. PACHECO E SILVA (1960-1961)
Professeur de psychiatrie à la Faculté de médecine de l'Université et de l'Ecole de médecine de Sao Paulo (Brésil)

GEORGE S. STEVENSON, M.D. (1961-1962)
Former National and International Consultant, National Association for Mental Health, Inc., New York

PHON SANGSINGKEO, M.D. (1962-1963)
Under-Secretary of State for Public Health, Ministry of Public Health, Bangkok

PROF. G.P. ALIVISATOS (1963-1964)
Professeur honoraire d'hygiène, Athènes

ALAN STOLLER, M.D. (1964-1965)
Chief Clinical Officer, Mental Hygiene Authority, Victoria (Australia)

CHIEF SIR SAMUEL MANUWA (1965-1966)
First Commissioner, Federal Public Service Commission, Lagos (Nigeria)

PROF. OTTO KLINEBERG (1966-1967)
International Center for Intergroup Relations, Paris, France

Rees the schemer, Répond the mental health-eugenist, Hoff the apologist and their cohorts.

From behind the Iron Curtain, Hegemann with the eugenists Palsvig, Ehrhardt, Répond and Pilkington.

From this list of names it is apparent to what degree the governments have been penetrated and infiltrated:
Director of a department in the Ministry of Health in Peru.
Director of the International Telecommunications Union (UN).
Chief of a section of the Ministry of Health in Venezuela.
Chief of a department of the Ministry of Health in Australia.
Head of a department of the Ministry of Education in Thailand.
Head of a department of the Ministry of Health in Egypt.
Director of the Mental Health Section of the World Health Organisation (former head of the World Health Organisation).
Under Secretary of State of Public Health in Bangkok.
Head of a department of the Ministry of Health in Australia.

Vorwort

Solange es unheilbar leidende, unter Schmerzen sterbende Menschen gibt, wird das Problem der „Euthanasie" zur Diskussion stehen. Die Organisation unseres modernen Lebens, die aus mancherlei Gründen Krankheit und Tod aus dem Familienbereich herausgerückt hat, mag vielen die willkommene Möglichkeit bieten, die hier aufbrechenden Fragen zu verdrängen. Damit hat man sie aber noch nicht aus der Welt geschafft und nur der Arzt, der sich ihnen am Sterbebett seiner Patienten nicht entziehen kann, wird in seinen Entscheidungen allein gelassen. Die „Verdrängung" des Euthanasie-Problems hat ihre Gründe jedoch nicht nur in der — menschlich begreiflichen — Tendenz vieler unserer Mitbürger, das Leiden ihrer Angehörigen nicht in seiner ganzen Schrecklichkeit mitzuerleben und dazu eine verantwortliche Stellung zu beziehen: Das Wort „Euthanasie" weckt auch die Erinnerung an die Tötung Kranker oder Mißgebildeter während der nationalsozialistischen Machtperiode, die man nicht gerne ins Gedächtnis zurückruft. Deshalb geht man in der Regel all diesen Fragen aus dem Weg. Selbst dort, wo sie auf breiter Basis zu einem die Öffentlichkeit beschäftigenden Thema werden, wie etwa bei der Tötung mißgebildeter Neugeborener in jüngster Zeit, steht ihrer sachlichen Erörterung häufig die „unbewältigte Vergangenheit" im Wege. Deshalb wird auch bei solchen konkreten Fällen entweder ein Teil der Problematik einfach außer Acht gelassen oder sie werden sogar unter Verwischung der jeweiligen Sachlage zu Rechtfertigungsversuchen für die Schuld der Vergangenheit herangezogen.

Angesichts dieser Scheu, die Dinge beim Namen zu nennen und ihnen in die Augen zu sehen, wirkt eine umfassende und objektive Darstellung, wie Professor E h r h a r d t sie in diesem Buche gibt, befreiend: Indem er nicht nur zunächst die Begriffe klar umreißt, sondern auch den historischen Ablauf der „Vernichtung lebensunwerten Lebens" im Dritten Reich schildert, öffnet er den Weg zu einer Bewältigung dieser Vergangenheit, ohne die eine weitere ernste Auseinandersetzung mit den Problemen der ärztlichen Ethik einfach nicht möglich ist. Da E h r h a r d t der Vielschichtigkeit der hier zur Diskussion stehenden Fragen durch eine mehrdimensionale Betrachtungsweise Rechnung trägt, gewinnt seine Darstellung eine bisher auf diesem Gebiete nie zuvor erreichte Plastizität. Deshalb wird dieses Buch nicht nur dem Studenten und Arzt, der eben wegen der Scheu vor diesem Thema hier in seinen Entscheidungen allein gelassen wird, von großer Hilfe sein, sondern auch jeden, der sich ernstlich mit der menschlichen Existenz auseinandersetzt, zur verantwortlichen Stellungnahme auch diesen Fragen gegenüber aufrufen.

Prof. Dr. H a n s H o f f
Vorstand der Psychiatrisch-Neurologischen
Universitätsklinik Wien

Hoff's preface to the book "Euthanasia and the Destruction of 'Life Unworthy' Life" by Helmut Ehrhardt.

Translation of Dr. Hoff's Foreword

[Editor: As Bernhard Schreiber did not translate this for his book, we have commissioned a translation ourselves, which was provided by Dr. Kirk Allison. This translation is copyrighted, and cannot be reproduced without permission.]

As long as there are incurably suffering people dying in pain the problem of "euthanasia" will be a topic of discussion. The organization of our modern life, which for various reasons has removed sickness and death from the familial realm, may offer to many the welcome possibility to repress questions raised here. However with that one has not yet removed them from the world and only the doctor, who cannot extract himself at the deathbed of his patients, is left in his decisions alone. The "repression" of the euthanasia problem has its reasons not only in the – humanly understandable – tendency of many of our fellow citizens to not experience the suffering of their relatives in its complete horror and take a responsible position to it: The word "euthanasia" awakens also the memory of the killing of sick or malformed during the National Socialist period of power which one does not gladly call back into memory. Therefore, as a rule, one avoids all of these questions. Even where they become a topic engaged by the public on a broad basis such as with the killing of malformed newborns in the most recent time the "unresolved past" stands in the way of its objective discussion. On that account in such concrete cases either a part of the problematic is simply left outside of consideration or they are even drawn upon under blurring of the respective circumstances for justificational attempts for the guilt of the past.

Given this reticence to name things by name and to look them in the eye, a comprehensive and objective depiction, as Professor Erhardt gives in this book, has a liberating effect: In that he not only initially clearly outlines the concepts, but also depicts the historical sequence of the "destruction of life unworthy of life" in the Third Reich, he opens the path to a coming to terms with this past without which a further serious engagement with the problems of medical ethics is simply not possible. As Erhardt allows for complexity of the questions under discussion here through a multidimensional manner of consideration, his depiction attains a never heretofore achieved plasticity. Therefore this book will be a great help not only to the student and physician who on account of reticence before this topic are here left alone in their decisions but also appeal to those who seriously engage with questions of human existence, also for the responsible taking of a position opposite these questions.

Prof. Dr. Hans Hoff
Directorate of the Psychiatric Neurological
University Clinic of Vienna

Published in 1962

THIS STATEMENT

is a revised and enlarged edition of

The Case for Voluntary Euthanasia (published in 1961)

———

It considers the new situation created by *The Suicide Act* (1961); and proposes a simplified plan for voluntary euthanasia, under safeguards which are thought to be appropriate.

*

It is presented by **The Euthanasia Society** with the approval of its President, The Rt. Hon. The Earl of Listowel, P.C., G.C.M.G., Ph.D., its Chairman, Dr. Leonard Colebrook, F.R.S., The Executive Committee, and of the following:

Mr. John Fortune.
Professor A. D. Gardner, D.M., F.R.C.S., F.R.C.P.
Mr. T. Gibson, F.R.C.S., F.R.F.P.S.
Dr. T. Howard Gillison, M.B., Ch.B.
Mr. Victor Gollancz, LL.D.
Rev. J. J. Goring, M.A., Ph.D.
Mr. R. S. Handley, O.B.E., F.R.C.S.
Professor C. H. Stuart Harris, C.B.E., M.D., F.R.C.P.
Mr. Jack Hawkins, C.B.E.
Rev. Joyce Hazlehurst, M.A., B.D.
Lord Henley.
Professor A. V. Hill, C.H., O.B.E., F.R.S.
Mrs. Margaret Hill, C.B.E.
Dr. Edward Hindle, F.R.S., Sc.D., Ph.D.
Rev. L. T. S. Hurn.
Mrs. Elspeth Huxley, C.B.E.
Elizabeth Jenkins.
Mr. Geoffrey Johnson.
Rev. Principal F. Kenworthy, M.A., B.D.
Mrs. Margaret Knight, M.A.
Captain B. H. Liddell-Hart.
Dr. Robert F. L. Logan, M.D., M.R.C.P.
Air Chief Marshal Sir Arthur Longmore, G.C.B., D.S.O.
Dr. E. J. L. Lowbury, M.A., D.M.
Sir Philip Manson-Bahr, C.M.G., D.S.O., M.D., F.R.C.P.
Dr. Ronald MacKeith, D.M., F.R.C.P.
Rev. H. J. McLachlan, M.A., B.D., D.Phil.
Dr. J. Maizel, L.R.C.S., L.R.C.P.
Mrs. C. I. Maizel, J.P.
Miss Ethel Mannin.
Sir John Maude, K.C.B., K.B.E.
Mr. W. Somerset Maugham, C.H., F.R.S.L.
Lady Mellanby, M.A., Sc.D.
Sir Frederick Messer, C.B.E., J.P.
Lady Milford.
Miss Phyllis Neilson-Terry.
Professor Wilfrid Newcomb, M.D., F.R.C.P.
Professor P. N. Nowell-Smith, M.A.
Dr. R. R. Race, F.R.S., Ph.D., F.R.C.P.
Rev. R. F. Rattray, M.A., Ph.D.
Miss Margaret Rawlings.
Dr. W. Ritchie Russell, M.D., D.Sc., F.R.C.P.
Mr. D. Kilham Roberts, O.B.E., M.A.
Miss Muriel Robertson, F.R.S., M.A., D.Sc.
Professor Dorothy Russell, M.D., Sc.D., LL.D., F.R.C.P.
Sir Harold Scott, G.C.V.O., K.C.B., K.B.E.
Mr. J. W. Robertson Scott.
Professor H. J. Seddon, C.M.G., F.R.C.S.

The supporters of voluntary euthanasia in 1961.

LIST OF PROMINENT SUPPORTERS OF "A PLEA FOR VOLUNTARY EUTHANASIA"

The Dowager Lady Aberconway
Lord Ailwyn, C.B.E.
G. B. Anderson, M.B.E., M.C., C.St.J.
Sir Christopher H. Andrewes, F.R.S., F.R.C.P., M.D., LL.D.
Dame Peggy Ashcroft, D.B.E., Hon.D.Litt.
John R. Baker, F.R.S., M.A., D.Sc., Ph.D.
Lord Balerno, C.B.E., D.Sc., F.R.S.E.
Lord Beaumont of Whitley
The Rt. Hon. Sir John Beaumont, P.C., Q.C.
Edward B. Benjamin
G. C. L. Bertram, M.A., Ph.D., F.I.Biol.
Aleck W. Bourne, M.A., M.B., B.Ch., F.R.C.S., F.R.C.O.G.
Professor C. D. Broad, M.A., Litt.D., F.B.A.
Lord Broughshane
Lord Brown, M.B.E.
Lady Marjorie Brown
Sir Felix Brunner, Bt.
Professor W. J. H. Butterfield, O.B.E., D.M., F.R.C.P.
Laurence J. Cadbury, O.B.E., M.A.
Professor C. A. Campbell, Hon.D.Litt.
H. J. Channon, C.M.G., D.Sc., F.R.I.C.
Lord Chorley, Q.C., J.P.
Dr. D. H. Clark, M.D., F.R.C.P.Edin., D.P.M.
Professor J. Patrick Corbett, M.A.
Dr. Saul Crown
Donald M. Douglas, M.D., F.R.C.P.Lond & Edin., D.C.H.
Professor Antony G. N. Flew
John Fortune
Professor O. R. Frisch, O.B.E., F.R.S., D.Sc.
Dr. T. Howard Gillison, M.B., M.R.C.P.
Sir Alister Hardy, M.A., D.Sc., F.R.S.
Lord Henley
Professor A. V. Hill, C.H., O.B.E., F.R.S., Sc.D., LL.D.
Dr. E. V. Hindle, F.R.S., Sc.D.
Professor Lancelot Hogben, F.R.S., M.A., D.Sc., LL.D.
The Earl of Huntingdon, M.A.
Elspeth Huxley, C.B.E., J.P.
Jill Hyem
Sir Christopher Ingold, F.R.S., D.Sc.
Elizabeth Jenkins
Rev. Principal F. Kenworthy, M.A., B.D.
The Earl Kitchener, T.D.
Ernest G. Kleinwort
Margaret Knight

Arthur Koestler, M.Inst.P.I., F.R.S.L.
Professor Hyman Levy, M.A., D.Sc., F.R.S.E.
W. Bennett Lewis, C.C., C.B.E., Ph.D., D.Sc., LL.D., F.
Brigadier Sir Clinton Lewis, O.B.E.
R. J. McNeill Love, M.S., F.R.C.S., F.A.C.S.
Dr. R. C. MacKeith, D.M., F.R.C.P., D.C.H.
Professor Donald M. MacKinnon, D.D.
The Rev. H. J. McLachlan, M.A., B.D., D.Phil.
Ethel Mannin
The Very Rev. W. R. Mathews, K.C.V.O., C.H., D.D., D
Lady Mellanby, M.A., Sc.D.
Lord Merthyr, P.C., K.B.E., T.D.
Dr. M. L. Millard
Professor Wilfrid D. Newcomb, M.D., F.R.C.P..
Peter Nichols
Sir W. Guy Nott-Bower, K.B.E., C.B.
Lady Paterson
Sir Robert Perkins
Dr. R. R. Race, F.R.S., F.R.C.P., Ph.D.
Margaret Rawlings
Dr. Mary M. Rayner
Professor Joseph Rotblat, C.B.E., D.Sc., F.Inst.P.
Professor Dorothy S. Russell, M.D., Sc.D., LL.D., F.R.
Dr. R. C. Sanders, M.A., B.M., B.Ch., M.R.C.P., D.M.R
Sir George Schuster, K.C.S.I., K.C.M.G., C.B.E., M.C.
Sir Herbert Seddon, C.M.G., D.M., LL.D., F.R.C.S.
The Hon. Lady Shuckberg
Lady Simon of Wythenshawe
Dr. Eliot Slater, C.B.E., M.D., F.R.C.P., D.P.M.
Ian M. Stephens, M.A.(Cantab.).
Dr. S. L. Henderson Smith
Lady Stocks, B.Sc.(Econ.), LL.D., Litt.D.
Lady Stokes, K.-i-H., M.A., M.R.C.S., L.R.C.P.
Viscount Stuart of Findhorn, P.C., C.H.
Lady Elizabeth Swann
Professor J. W. Tibble, M.A., M.Ed.
Professor John Walton, Sc.D., Dr.-es-Sc., LL.D., F.R.S.
The Rev. Leslie C. Weatherhead, C.B.E., M.A., Ph.D,
  D.Litt., D.D.
The Rev. D. G. Wigmore-Beddoes, M.A., F.R.S.A.
Professor Glanville Williams, Q.C., F.B.A., LL.D.
His Grace the Duke of Wellington
The Rt. Rev. J. L. Wilson (formerly Bishop of Birming
  K.C.M.G., M.A., D.D., D.Sc.

The supporters of voluntary euthanasia in 1971.
Felix Brunner, D. H. Clark, Eliot Slater, Lady Stocks, Profes
Williams.
They are all strong forces in the mental health movement.

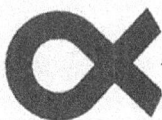

The supporters of abortion reform 1969-1970.
Viscountess Monckton, Lady Stocks, Julian Huxley, Prof. Carstairs,
Eliot Slater.

Birth Control Campaign

president
The Rt Hon the Lord Gardiner

vice presidents
Mrs Vera Houghton
Mrs Lena Jeger MP
The Rt Hon Lord Molson
The Baroness Serota JP
Sir George Sinclair CMG OBE MP
David M S Steel MA LLB MP

advisory council
Professor Brian Abel-Smith MA PhD (Cantab)
J A Banks MA
The Baroness Birk JP
The Rt Hon Lord Boyle of Handsworth
Mrs Helen Brook
Edwin Brooks MA PhD
The Lord Burntwood
Mrs Barbara Cadbury
C O Carter MA DM FRCP
The Rt Hon R H S Crossman OBE MP
Peter Diggory FRCS MRCOG
The Baroness Gaitskell
The Rev Dr Kenneth Greet
Professor Peter Huntingford MD FRCOG
Mrs Stephanie Kerans
Professor Ian MacGillivray MD FRCOG
The Dowager Viscountess Monckton of
    Brenchley CBE
Professor Norman Morris MD FRCOG
Rt Hon Sir David Renton KBE TD QC MP
The Rt Rev Dr J A T Robinson
Michael Schofield MA
Sir Frederic Seebohm TD
The Rt Hon the Earl of Selkirk
    GCMG GBE AFC QC
Eliot Slater CBE MD FRCP DPM
The Rev the Lord Soper MA PhD
The Baroness Stocks BSc
Professor Glanville Williams QC LLD FBA

management committee
Alastair Service/chairman
Paul M Dayton FCA/treasurer
D P Christine Beazley
Enid Binks
Juliet Carpenter
Dr John Dunwoody
Stanley Johnson
Margot Pearson
Dr D Malcolm Potts
Caroline Woodroffe

general secretary Dilys Cossey
Birth Control Campaign
233 Tottenham Court Road
London W1P 9AE
Tel: 01-580 9360

The supporters of Birth Control Campaign.
R. H. S. Crossman, Viscountess Monckton, Eliot Slater, Baroness
Stocks, Prof. Williams.

Die Stellung des Nationalsozialismus zur Rassenhygiene.

Von Prof. F. Lenz, München.

Die Nationalsozialistische Deutsche Arbeiterpartei (N.S.D.A.P.) ist die erste politische Partei, nicht nur in Deutschland, sondern überhaupt, welche die Rassenhygiene als eine zentrale Forderung ihres Programms vertritt. Das ist um so bemerkenswerter, als sie aus den Wahlen vom September 1930 mit 107 Mandaten als zweitstärkste Partei des Deutschen Reichstags hervorgegangen ist. Sie ist dabei grundsätzlich antiparlamentarisch eingestellt; und ihre eigentliche Bedeutung liegt demgemäß nicht in der nationalsozialistischen Reichstagsfraktion, sondern in der von ihr getragenen politischen Bewegung, die in den nächsten Jahren voraussichtlich von großem Einfluß auf die innere und äußere Politik des Deutschen Reiches sein wird. Das ist für mich der Grund, weshalb ich mich hier mit der Stellung der nationalsozialistischen Bewegung zur Rassenhygiene befasse.

Ich stütze mich in meinem Bericht hauptsächlich auf das Buch Adolf Hitlers*), der als Begründer der nationalsozialistischen Bewegung anzusehen ist und der auch gegenwärtig ihr maßgebender Führer ist. Hitler ist als Sohn eines Zollbeamten bayerischen Stammes, aber österreichischer Staatsangehörigkeit, in Braunau am Inn geboren und gegenwärtig einige vierzig Jahre alt. Nach dem Tode seines Vaters mußte er sich in jungen Jahren als Hilfsarbeiter durchschlagen. Sein Ziel war, Baumeister zu werden. Nachdem er in der Jugend mehrere Jahre in Wien gearbeitet hatte, siedelte er 1912 nach München über.

------

*) Hitler, A., Mein Kampf. 782 S. 5. Aufl. München 1930. Verlag Franz Eher.

Den Weltkrieg hat er als Frontkämpfer in einem bayerischen Regiment mitgemacht. Seit der deutschen Revolution hat er sich dann ganz der Politik gewidmet. Dank einer ganz außergewöhnlichen Fähigkeit der Massenbeeinflussung gelang es ihm, in den Jahren 1920 bis 1923 Hunderttausende von national begeisterten Anhängern, meist jungen Leuten, zu gewinnen. Im November 1923 glaubte er die Stunde für eine nationale Gegenrevolution und Erhebung gekommen. Die Bewegung wurde aber durch Machtmittel des Staates unterdrückt und Hitler zu einer mehrjährigen Festungshaft verurteilt. In dieser Zeit hat er sein Buch geschrieben.

In dem Kapitel „Der Staat" bemerkt Hitler im Hinblick auf die Rassenhygiene: „Was auf diesem Gebiete heute von allen Seiten versäumt wird, hat der völkische Staat nachzuholen. Er hat die Rasse in den Mittelpunkt des allgemeinen Lebens zu setzen" (S. 446). Ja, das soll sogar der eigentliche Zweck des Staates sein: „Sein Zweck liegt in der Erhaltung und Förderung einer Gemeinschaft physisch und seelisch gleichartiger Lebewesen. Diese Erhaltung selber umfaßt erstlich den rassenmäßigen Bestand und gestattet dadurch die freie Entwicklung aller in dieser Rasse schlummernden Kräfte" (S. 433). Ein Staat, der die rassische Grundlage der Kultur dem Untergange weiht, muß als schlecht bezeichnet werden (S. 435).

Der Staat muß nach Hitler dafür sorgen, daß nur gesunde Menschen Kinder zeugen. „Wer körperlich und geistig nicht gesund und würdig ist, darf sein Leid nicht im Körper seines Kindes verewigen." „Umgekehrt aber muß es als verwerflich gelten: gesunde Kinder der Nation vorzuenthalten. Der Staat muß dabei als Wahrer einer tausendjährigen Zukunft auftreten, der gegenüber der Wunsch und die Eigensucht des einzelnen als nichts erscheinen und sich zu beugen haben. Er hat die modernsten ärztlichen Hilfsmittel in den Dienst dieser Erkenntnis zu stellen. Er hat, was irgendwie ersichtlich krank und erblich belastet und damit weiter belastend ist, zeugungsunfähig zu erklären und dies praktisch auch durchzusetzen. Er hat umgekehrt dafür zu sorgen, daß die Fruchtbarkeit des gesunden Weibes nicht beschränkt wird durch die finanzielle Luderwirtschaft eines Staatsregiments, das den Kindersegen zu einem Fluch für die Eltern gestaltet" (S. 447). Hitler fordert also einen Ausgleich der Familienlasten, wenn er auch diesen Ausdruck nicht gebraucht. „Der völkische Staat hat hier die ungeheuerste Erziehungsarbeit zu leisten. Sie wird aber dereinst auch als eine größere Tat erscheinen, als es die siegreichsten Kriege unseres heutigen bürgerlichen Zeitalters sind" (S. 447). Der Staat müsse „ohne Rücksicht auf Verständnis oder Unverständnis, Billigung oder Mißbilligung in diesem Sinne handeln".

Natürlich sind es nicht neue Ideen, die Hitler hier vertritt. Aus welchen Quellen er geschöpft hat, hat er nicht angegeben, vermutlich mit bewußter Absicht; denn ein wissenschaftliches Werk mit Quellenbelegen hat nun einmal nicht eine politische Massenwirkung, wie sie ein Schriftsteller erreichen kann, der im Stile des Propheten schreibt. Einige Wendungen erinnern an Äußerungen Nietzsches, der im „Willen zur Macht" Absatz 734 u. a. sagt: „Es gibt Fälle, wo ein Kind ein Verbrechen sein würde." „Zuletzt hat hier die Gesellschaft eine Pflicht zu erfüllen: es gibt wenige dergestalt dringliche und grundsätzliche Forderungen an sie. Die Gesellschaft als Großmandatar des Lebens hat jedes verfehlte Leben vor dem Leben selber zu verantworten, — sie hat es auch zu büßen: folglich soll sie es verhindern. Die Gesellschaft soll in zahlreichen Fällen der Zeugung vorbeugen: sie darf hierzu, ohne Rücksicht auf Herkunft, Rang und Geist, die härtesten Zwangsmaßregeln, Freiheitsentziehungen, unter Umständen Kastrationen in Bereitschaft halten." Von eigentlich rassenhygienischen Büchern hat Hitler, wie ich höre, die zweite Auflage des Baur-Fischer-Lenz gelesen, und zwar während seiner Festungshaft in Landsberg. Manche Stellen daraus spiegeln sich in Wendungen Hitlers wieder. Jedenfalls hat er die wesentlichen Gedanken der Rassenhygiene und ihre Bedeutung mit großer geistiger Empfänglichkeit und Energie sich zu eigen gemacht, während die meisten akademischen Autoritäten diesen Fragen noch ziemlich verständnislos gegenüberstehen. Es ist überhaupt erstaunlich, wie Hitler, der nur eine Realschule besucht hat, sich unter schwierigen Verhältnissen durch privates Bücherstudium jene Bildung hat aneignen können, die aus seinem Buche spricht. Über die Möglichkeiten der Rassenhygiene urteilt er zusammenfassend folgendermaßen: „Eine nur sechshundertjährige Verhinderung der Zeugungsfähigkeit und Zeugungsmöglichkeit seitens körperlich Degenerierter und geistig Erkrankter würde die Menschheit nicht nur von einem unermeßlichen Unglück befreien, sondern zu einer Gesundung beitragen, die heute kaum faßbar erscheint. Wenn so die bewußte planmäßige Förderung der Fruchtbarkeit der gesündesten Träger des Volkstums verwirklicht wird, so wird das Ergebnis eine Rasse sein, die, zunächst wenigstens, die Keime unseres heutigen körperlichen und damit auch geistigen Verfalls wieder ausgeschieden haben wird" (S. 448). Die einschränkenden Worte „zunächst wenigstens" sollen offenbar besagen, daß die Gesundung der Erbmasse des Volkes die nächste und dringendste Aufgabe ist. Darüber hinaus aber hält Hitler auch die Förderung besonders hochwertiger rassischer Elemente für angezeigt. Er meint: „Denn hat erst ein Volk und Staat diesen Weg einmal beschritten, dann wird sich auch von selbst das Augenmerk darauf richten, gerade den rassisch wertvollsten Kern des Volkes und gerade seine Fruchtbarkeit zu steigern, um endlich das gesamte Volkstum des Segens eines hochgezüchteten Rassengutes teilhaftig werden zu lassen" (S. 448, ähnlich auch S. 493). „Ein Staat, der im Zeitalter der Rassenvergiftung sich der Pflege seiner besten rassischen Elemente widmet, muß eines Tages zum Herrn der Erde werden" (S. 782).

Hitler hat anscheinend auch eine besondere Förderung nordischer Rassenelemente im Auge. Der Begriff „Nordische Rasse" kommt zwar, soviel ich sehe, in dem Buche nicht vor; an zahlreichen Stellen preist er aber die „Arier", denen er als Gegenpol die Juden gegenüberstellt. Die Juden werden — zweifellos zu einseitig und in übertriebener Weise — für fast alle Zersetzungserscheinungen der Gegenwart verantwortlich gemacht. Dem Juden fehlen nach Hitler „jene Eigenschaften, die schöpferisch und damit kulturell begnadete Rassen auszeichnen"; sie besitzen „keine irgendwie kulturbildende Kraft" (S. 332). Die Vortrefflichkeit des „Ariers" erstrahlt im Vergleich zu diesem dunklen Hintergrunde in um so hellerem Licht. „Alles, was wir heute auf dieser Erde bewundern — Wissenschaft und Kunst, Technik und Erfindungen —, ist nur das schöpferische Produkt weniger Völker und vielleicht ursprünglich einer Rasse. Von ihnen hängt auch der Bestand dieser ganzen Kultur ab. Gehen sie zugrunde, so sinkt mit ihnen die Schönheit dieser Erde ins Grab." „Alle großen Kulturen der Vergangenheit gingen nur zugrunde, weil die ursprünglich schöpferische Rasse an Blutsvergiftung abstarb" (S. 316). „Die Rassenfrage gibt nicht nur den Schlüssel zur Weltgeschichte, sondern auch zur menschlichen Kultur überhaupt" (S. 372). Hitler ist offenbar stark von H. St. Chamberlain beeinflußt worden, indirekt vielleicht auch von Gobineau, der zwar auch die Juden nicht liebte, ihnen aber doch mehr gerecht wurde. Auch von Th. Fritsch hat er anscheinend manche Ansichten übernommen. Ein Einfluß Günthers auf Hitlers Buch ist weniger deutlich; doch ist anzunehmen, daß er auch Günther gelesen hat.

Wie Gobineau und Chamberlain übertreibt Hitler die schädlichen Folgen der Rassenkreuzung. „Die Blutsvermischung und das dadurch bedingte Senken des Rassenniveaus ist die alleinige Ursache des Absterbens alter Kulturen; denn die Menschen gehen nicht an verlorenen Kriegen zugrunde, sondern am Verlust jener Widerstandskraft, die nur dem reinen Blute zu eigen ist" (S. 324, ähnlich auch S. 442 und 443). An anderen Stellen zeigt er freilich auch Verständnis für die Hemmung der Auslese als Entartungsursache (z. B. S. 145) und für die wirklich entscheidende Ursache des Niedergangs, die Gegenauslese, z. B. auf S. 582 und 583, wo er von der Auslesewirkung des Krieges spricht. Die grundlegende Bedeutung der Auslese für die Gestaltung der Rassen und Arten wird auf S. 144/145 und S. 313 betont.

An sich ist es gewiß richtig, daß die Rassenhygiene sich die Erhaltung und Förderung jener Rassenelemente, die unsere Kultur geschaffen haben, angelegen sein lassen muß. „Somit ist der höchste Zweck des völkischen Staates die Sorge um die Erhaltung derjenigen rassischen Urelemente, die, als kulturspendend, die Schönheit und Würde eines höheren Menschentums schaffen" (S. 434). Es kommt aber sehr darauf an, wie „der Versuch, die innerhalb der Volksgemeinschaft als rassisch besonders wertvoll erkannten Elemente maßgeblichst zu fördern und für ihre besondere Vermehrung Sorge zu tragen" (S. 493), praktisch durchzuführen gesucht wird. Hitler denkt an Siedlungskolonien, „deren Bewohner ausschließlich Träger höchster Rassenreinheit und damit höchster Rassentüchtigkeit sind" (S. 449). „Eigens gebildete Rassekommissionen haben den einzelnen das Siedlungsattest auszustellen; dieses aber ist gebunden an eine festzulegende bestimmte rassische Reinheit" (S. 448). Nun ist es aber in einer gemischten Bevölkerung wie der unsrigen nicht möglich, nach äußeren Merkmalen die Zugehörigkeit des wesentlichen Teils der Erbmasse festzustellen. Blondes Haar verbürgt nicht edle Rasse und dunkles schließt sie nicht aus. In bezug auf die soziale Auslese bemerkt Hitler treffend: „Diese Siebung nach Fähigkeit und Tüchtigkeit kann nicht mechanisch vorgenommen werden, sondern ist eine Arbeit, die der Kampf des täglichen Lebens ununterbrochen besorgt" (S. 493). Diese Bewährung im täglichen Leben ist meines Erachtens auch der beste Maßstab für die rassenhygienische Auslese. Natürlich darf auch nicht etwa das Parteibuch als Maßstab der Tüchtigkeit genommen werden. Ein Beispiel rassischen Niedergangs ist für Hitler das ihm auch sonst unsympathische Frankreich. Dieses macht nach Hitler „in seiner Vernegerung so rapide Fortschritte, daß man tatsächlich von einer Entstehung eines afrikanischen Staates auf europäischem Boden reden kann" (S. 730). Mag das auch übertrieben erscheinen, die Gefahr,

welche direkt für Frankreich und indirekt für ganz Europa droht, ist doch grundsätzlich richtig gesehen. Wenn er von dem „nicht nur in seiner Volkszahl, sondern
besonders in seinen rassisch besten Elementen absterbenden Franzosentum"
spricht (S. 766), so scheint er allerdings bei der Niederschrift dieses Satzes sich
nicht bewußt gewesen zu sein, daß die gegenwärtige Kinderzahl des deutschen
Volkes noch weniger zur Erhaltung ausreicht als die des französischen.

Hitler setzt sich energisch für die Sterilisierung Minderwertiger ein. „Die
Forderung, daß defekten Menschen die Zeugung anderer ebenso defekter Nachkommen unmöglich gemacht wird, ist eine Forderung klarster Vernunft und
bedeutet in ihrer planmäßigen Durchführung die humanste Tat der Menschheit.
Sie wird Millionen von Unglücklichen unverdiente Leiden ersparen, in der Folge
aber zu einer steigenden Gesundung überhaupt führen" (S. 279). Aus der Tat-
sache, daß er von Millionen von Unglücklichen spricht, folgt, daß er die Sterilisierung nicht nur für extreme Fälle fordert, was für die Gesundung der Rasse
ziemlich bedeutungslos sein würde, sondern sie auf den gesamten minderwertigen Teil der Bevölkerung erstreckt wissen will.

Er weiß auch die Bedeutung früher Eheschließung in ihrer ganzen Tragweite
zu würdigen. „Freilich ist zu ihrer Ermöglichung eine ganze Reihe von sozialen
Voraussetzungen nötig, ohne die an eine frühe Verehelichung gar nicht zu denken ist" (S. 276). Er sieht durchaus ein, daß eine Lösung dieser Frage nicht ohne
einschneidende soziale Maßnahmen möglich ist. Man darf also hoffen, daß die
nationalsozialistische Bewegung sich tatkräftig für einen Ausgleich der Familienlasten einsetzen wird.

Treffend sind auch die Bemerkungen über die Steigerung der Lebensansprüche,
die eine Hauptursache übermäßiger Geburtenbeschränkung ist. „Die Anforde-
rungen der Menschen in bezug auf Nahrung und Kleidung werden von Jahr zu
Jahr größer und stehen schon jetzt zum Beispiel in keinem Verhältnis mehr zu
den Bedürfnissen unserer Vorfahren etwa vor 100 Jahren" (S. 146). Da die Steigerung der Ansprüche zum guten Teil durch den Aufwand der Kinderlosen bedingt
ist, würde ein wirksamer Ausgleich der Familienlasten, die übermäßige Steigerung der Ansprüche zurückzuschrauben geeignet sein. „Sicherlich wird zu einem
bestimmten Zeitpunkt die gesamte Menschheit gezwungen sein, infolge der Un-
möglichkeit, die Fruchtbarkeit des Bodens der weitersteigenden Volkszahl noch
länger anzugleichen, die Vermehrung des menschlichen Geschlechts einzu-
stellen" (S. 147). Einem Volk, das mit der Einstellung der Fortpflanzung voran-
geht, wird aber das Dasein auf dieser Welt genommen (S. 145).

Eine wichtige Voraussetzung für die Erhaltung der rassenmäßigen Grundlagen unseres Volkstums ist eine in diesem Sinne gestaltete Erziehung. „Die gesamte Bildungs- und Erziehungsarbeit des völkischen Staates muß ihre Krönung
darin finden, daß sie den Rassesinn und das Rassegefühl instinkt- und verstan-
desmäßig in Herz und Gehirn der ihr anvertrauten Jugend hineinbrennt" (S. 475).
„Das Ziel der weiblichen Erziehung hat unverrückbar die kommende Mutter zu
sein" (S. 460). Das jugendliche Gehirn soll im allgemeinen nicht mit Dingen belastet werden, die es zu 95 Prozent nicht braucht (S. 464). Der französische
Sprachunterricht sollte von den höheren Schulen entfernt werden (S. 465). Im
Geschichtsunterricht sollte eine wesentliche Kürzung des Stoffes vorgenommen

werden (S. 467); in der Geschichte kommt der Rassenfrage die dominierende Stellung zu (S. 468). Wenn der überflüssige und daher schädliche Bildungswust von der Schule entfernt werden würde, so würde, wie ich hinzufügen möchte, es auch möglich sein, die gesamte Dauer der höheren Schule um zwei Jahre zu kürzen, was im Hinblick auf die Ermöglichung früherer Eheschließung dringend erwünscht wäre.

Eine ebenso wichtige Aufgabe des Bildungswesens, wie die Erziehung es ist, ist die soziale Auslese oder, wie Hitler sich ausdrückt, „die Menschenauslese an sich" (S. 477). Der völkische Staat hat „nicht die Aufgabe, einer bestehenden Gesellschaftsklasse den maßgebenden Einfluß zu wahren, sondern die Aufgabe, aus der Summe aller Volksgenossen die fähigsten Köpfe herauszuholen und zu Amt und Würden zu bringen" (S. 480). Der Rassenhygieniker muß aber darauf dringen, daß die fähigen Köpfe nicht wie bisher eben durch ihren Aufstieg dem Aussterben zugeführt werden. Hitler ist der Gedanke unerträglich, „daß alljährlich Hunderttausende vollständig talentlose Menschen einer höheren Ausbildung gewürdigt werden, während andere Hunderttausende von großer Begabung ohne jede höhere Ausbildung bleiben" (S. 479). Über die Häufigkeit hoher geistiger Begabung in den unteren Schichten scheint sich Hitler allerdings zu optimistische Vorstellungen zu machen. Hier wäre auf die Feststellungen Hartnackes hinzuweisen (Naturgrenzen geistiger Bildung, Leipzig 1930).

Im übrigen scheut Hitler sich nicht, auch unpopuläre Wahrheiten auszusprechen. So bemerkt er zur Alkoholfrage: „Wenn z. B. ein ganzer Kontinent der Alkoholvergiftung endlich den Kampf ansagt, um ein Volk aus den Klammern dieses verheerenden Lasters herauszulösen, dann hat unsere europäische bürgerliche Welt dafür nichts übrig als ein nichtssagendes Glotzen und Kopfschütteln, ein überlegenes Lächerlichfinden — das sich bei dieser lächerlichen Gesellschaft besonders gut ausnimmt" (S. 450). Auch sonst nennt er die Dinge oft beim rechten Namen: „Unser gesamtes öffentliches Leben gleicht heute einem Treibhaus sexueller Vorstellungen und Reize. Man betrachte doch den Speisezettel unserer Kinos, Varietés und Theater, und man kann wohl kaum leugnen, daß dies nicht die richtige Kost, vor allem für die Jugend, ist" (S. 278).

Auch die Außenpolitik muß das Ziel haben, „die Existenz der durch den Staat zusammengefaßten Rasse sicherzustellen" (S. 728). Wenn Deutschland im Jahre 1904 die Rolle Japans übernommen hätte, so wäre einem Weltkriege vorgebeugt gewesen. „Das Blut im Jahre 1904 hätte das zehnfache der Jahre 1914 bis 1918 erspart" (S. 155). Dazu war die Freundschaft Englands nötig. Es war daher auf Kolonien und Seegeltung zu verzichten; die gesamten Machtmittel des Staates waren auf das Landheer zu konzentrieren (S. 154, ähnlich auch S. 753). Der sogenannte „Risikogedanke" von Tirpitz wird als grundfalsch bezeichnet (S. 300). „Ich gestehe offen, daß ich schon in der Vorkriegszeit es für richtiger gehalten hätte, wenn sich Deutschland, unter Verzicht auf die unsinnige Kolonialpolitik und unter Verzicht auf Handels- und Kriegsflotte, mit England im Bunde gegen Rußland gestellt hätte und damit von der schwachen Allerweltspolitik zu einer entschlossenen europäischen Politik kontinentalen Bodenerwerbs übergegangen wäre" (S. 753). Ich kann diesen Ausführungen nur zustimmen; und ich habe mich verschiedentlich im gleichen Sinne geäußert (z. B. B.-F.-L. Bd. II S. 396/397).

Hitler glaubt, daß eine solche Politik auch in Zukunft wieder möglich sein werde;
und er möchte in diesem Sinne dem deutschen Volk ein „politisches Testament"
geben, ein großes Ziel, an dem die Außenpolitik unbeschadet der etwa nötigen
Entscheidungen des Tages zu orientieren sei. „Wir stoppen den ewigen Germanen-
zug nach dem Süden und Westen Europas und weisen den Blick nach dem Land
im Osten. Wir schließen endlich ab die Kolonial- und Handelspolitik der Vorkriegszeit und gehen über zur Bodenpolitik der Zukunft" (S. 742). Die Entwicklung der Weltwirtschaft in den Jahren, seit Hitler dies geschrieben hat, weist
unser Volk in die gleiche Richtung. Wir werden einfach gezwungen sein, unsere
Lebensgrundlage wieder vorwiegend auf dem Lande zu suchen. „Schon die Möglichkeit eines gesunden Bauernstandes als Fundament der gesamten Nation kann
niemals hoch genug eingeschätzt werden. Viele unserer heutigen Leiden sind
nur die Folge des ungesunden Verhältnisses zwischen Land- und Stadtvolk"
(S. 157).

Aus einer solchen Politik würde sich auch ganz von selbst eine Interessen-
gemeinschaft der großen germanischen Völker ergeben, die nicht nur aus ideellen
Gründen anzustreben ist, sondern die aus dem wohlverstandenen Lebensinter-
esse der einzelnen germanischen Völker folgt. „Man darf sich nicht durch Ver-
schiedenheiten der einzelnen Völker die größere Rassegemeinschaft zerreißen
lassen. Der Kampf, der heute tobt, geht um ganz große Ziele: eine Kultur kämpft
um ihr Dasein, die Jahrtausende in sich verbindet und Griechen- und Germanen-
tum gemeinsam umschließt" (S. 470).

Hitler wendet sich scharf gegen die Forderung der Wiederherstellung der
deutschen Grenzen von 1914, die er als einen politischen Unsinn von Ausmaßen
und Folgen bezeichnet, die ihn als Verbrechen erscheinen lassen. Auch abgesehen
von dem Umstande, daß zu einer solchen Politik die Machtmittel fehlen, würde
sie, selbst wenn sie erfolgreich wäre, zu einer weiteren Ausblutung unseres Volks-
körpers führen, die nicht verantwortet werden könnte (S. 739). Insbesondere auf
Südtirol muß ganz bewußt verzichtet werden, da wir die Freundschaft Italiens
ebensowenig wie die Englands entbehren können. Im Hinblick auf die Möglichkeit künftiger Kriege sagt Hitler: „Eine Diplomatie hat dafür zu sorgen, daß
ein Volk nicht heroisch zugrunde geht, sondern praktisch erhalten wird" (S. 693).
„Wir schwärmen auch heute noch von einem Heroismus, der unserem Volke
Millionen seiner edelsten Blutträger raubte, im Endergebnis jedoch vollkommen
unfruchtbar blieb" (S. 735). Heute vollends seien die Machtmittel des Deutschen
Reiches so jämmerlich, daß ein Kampf gegen Frankreich nur den Charakter eines
„Abschlachtens der deutschen Jugend haben würde; und das Endergebnis wäre
die unabwendbare Niederlage und das Ende des Deutschen Reiches.

In einem künftigen Kriege wird die technische Rüstung mehr als die Zahl der
Soldaten entscheidend sein (S. 748). Durch diesen Satz wird gewissermaßen ein
früherer richtiggestellt, in dem Hitler von der Wiedergewinnung äußerer Macht
sagt: „Die Voraussetzungen hierzu sind aber nicht, wie unsere bürgerlichen
‚Staatsmänner' immer herumschwätzen, Waffen, sondern Kräfte des Willens"
(S. 365). In dieser Hinsicht haben die „bürgerlichen" Staatsmänner eben doch
nicht so unrecht gehabt. Und sie hatten insbesondere recht gegenüber dem
Hitler von 1923, der das vergessen hatte. Wenn Hitler damals größere An-

fangserfolge gehabt hätte, so hätte Frankreich sich die Gelegenheit zum Abschießen des Restes der deutschen Jugend nicht entgehen lassen und sein auch von Hitler als solches gekennzeichnetes Ziel erreicht, die Zerschlagung des Deutschen Reiches. Man kann es gewiß verstehen, daß Hitlers nationale Begeisterung ihn damals zu einem Schritte hingerissen hat, den er schwerlich getan hätte, wenn er „die Vernunft als alleinige Führerin" hätte gelten lassen, wie er auf S. 753 als Grundsatz ausspricht. Vermutlich weiß er heute selber, daß es für den Bestand des Reiches besser war, daß die Erhebung damals gleich in den Anfängen unterdrückt wurde. Gewiß muß ein Krebskranker eine Operation wagen, auch wenn nur ein halbes Prozent Aussicht auf Erfolg besteht (S. 463); Hitler selbst aber wird zugeben, daß die Aussichten auf Rettung von Reich und Volk heute besser sind als im Jahre 1923 und daß begründete Hoffnung besteht, daß sie noch besser werden. Und er selber hat heute und in Zukunft bessere Aussichten, an dieser Rettung wesentlich mitzuwirken als damals.

Hitlers Fähigkeit der suggestiven Beeinflussung von Massen ist bewundernswert. Über die Mittel und Wege der Massenbeeinflussung spricht er mit erstaunlicher Offenheit. „Die Propaganda ist in Inhalt und Form auf die breite Masse anzusetzen, und ihre Richtigkeit ist ausschließlich zu messen an ihrem wirksamen Erfolg" (S. 376). „Solange die Einsicht der Masse so gering bleibt wie jetzt und der Staat so gleichgültig wie heute, wird diese Masse stets dem am ersten folgen, der in wirtschaftlichen Dingen zunächst die unverschämtesten Versprechungen bietet" (S. 354). Gift werde nur durch Gegengift überwunden. Man darf annehmen, daß Hitler genau weiß, daß ein Volk auch von Gegengift nicht leben kann. „Die Rede eines Staatsmanns zu seinem Volk habe ich nicht zu messen nach dem Eindruck, den sie bei einem Universitätsprofessor hinterläßt, sondern an der Wirkung, die sie auf das Volk ausübt" (S. 534). Dieses Umstandes wird man stets eingedenk sein müssen, wenn man gewisse Auslassungen Hitlers über wirtschaftliche Forderungen, über Möglichkeiten der Außenpolitik und auch über die Judenfrage liest, über die man manchmal den Kopf schüttelt........... ...

The Relation of National Socialism to Racial Hygiene

By Prof. F. Lenz. Munich

The Nationalsozialistische Deutsche Arbeiterpartei (N.S.D.A.P.) is the first political party, not only in Germany, but generally, which supports racial hygiene as a central part of its platform. What is more remarkable, is that it emerged from the elections in September 1930 with 107 representatives as the second strongest party in the German Reichstag. It is essentially anti-parliamentarian, and therefore its actual significance lies not in the proportion of national socialists in the Reichstag, but in the political movement which it carries and which in the coming years will probably have a great deal of influence on the home and foreign policies of the German Reich. This is the reason why I deal with the relationship of the national socialist movement to racial hygiene at this point.

I base my report mainly on the book (**Mein Kampf**) of Adolf Hitler, who is to be regarded as the founder of the national socialist movement, and who is presently its decisive Führer. Hitler, the son of a customs-official of Bavarian stock but of Austrian nationality, was born in Braunau on the Inn. He is presently some forty years old. After the death of his father, he had to fight his way up as an unskilled labourer. It was his aim to become an architect. Having worked in Vienna in his youth for several years, he moved to Munich in 1912. In the first World War he was a soldier at the front in a Bavarian regiment. Since the German Revolution, he has devoted himself wholly to politics. Thanks to his exceptional ability in influencing the masses, in the years from 1920 to 1923 he succeeded in winning hundreds of thousands of nationalistic and enthusiastic followers, most of them young people. In November 1923, he thought that the hour for a national counter-revolution and uprising had come. However, this movement was suppressed by state force, and Hitler was sentenced to a prison term for some years. During this time, he wrote his book. In the chapter, "The State", Hitler commented on racial hygiene: "The folkish state must make up for what everyone else today has neglected in this field. It must put the race as the centre of all life." (P. 446). In fact, this must be the actual purpose of the state: "The end lies in the preservation and advancement of a community of physically and mentally homogenous creatures. This preservation itself comprises first of all existence as a race and thereby permits the free development of all the forces dormant in the race." (P. 433). A state can be designated as bad if it dooms the bearer of this culture by his racial composition. (P. 435).

The state, according to Hitler, must ensure that only the healthy beget children. "Those who are physically and mentally unhealthy and unworthy must not perpetuate their suffering in the bodies of their children." "And conversely it must be considered reprehensible to withhold healthy children from the nation. Here the state must act as the guardian of a millennial future, in the face of which the wishes and selfishness of the individual must become nothing and submit. It must declare unfit for propagation all who are in any way visibly sick or who have inherited a disease and can therefore pass it on, and it can put this into actual practice. Conversely, it must take care that the fertility of the healthy woman is not limited by the financial irresponsibility of a state regime which turns the blessing of children into a curse for the parents." (P. 477) In other words, Hitler demands compensation for family burdens, even if he does not use this expression. "In this the folkish state must perform the most gigantic educational task. And some day this will seem to be a greater deed than the most victorious wars of our present bourgeois era." (P. 447). The state "must act in this sense without regard to understanding or lack of understanding, approval or disapproval."

Naturally the ideas which Hitler advocates are not new. He did not mention the sources from which he drew, presumably with conscious intention, as a scientific work with source-references just does not have the political mass-effect of that of a writer who writes in the style of a prophet. Some of the expressions remind one of Nietzsche's comments, who says in "Will to Power" paragraph 734 amongst other things: "There are cases where a child would be a crime". "In the final analysis society has to perform a duty here: there are few more urgent and basic demands of this nature on a society. Society as a great authorized agent of life must be made responsible for every unsuccessful life — it has to pay for it, so it must prohibit it. Society should guard against many cases of procreation: for this it is permitted to keep in readiness — irrespective of origin, rank and class — the hardest coercive measures, penal sentences and possibly castration." Of the actual racial hygienic books Hitler read, so I am told, is the second edition of Baur-Fischer-Lenz. This was during his prison sentence in Landsberg. Some parts of it can be seen in the expressions of Hitler. In any case, he has taken the essential ideas of racial hygiene and its importance and enhanced them with a great mental receptiveness and energy of his own, whereas most of the academic authorities still stand quite unappreciative of these questions. In fact it is quite astounding that Hitler, who only went to high school, could under these difficult conditions acquire through private study the education which emerges from his book. Concerning the possibilities of racial hygiene, he judges summarily as follows: "A prevention of the faculty and opportunity to procreate on the part of the physically degenerate and mentally sick over a period of only six hundred years, would not only free humanity from an immeasurable misfortune, but would lead to a recovery which today seems scarcely conceivable. If the fertility of the healthiest bearers of nationality is thus consciously and systematically promoted, the result will be a race which in the meantime at least will have eliminated the germs of our present physical and hence spiritual decay." The limiting words "in the meantime at least" are obviously intended to indicate that the recovery of hereditary mass is the next and most vital task. Also Hitler deems the demand for especially high grade racial elements to be advisable. He thinks: "For once a people and a state have started on this path, attention will automatically be directed toward increasing the racially most valuable nucleus of the race and its fertility, in order ultimately to let the entire nationality partake of the blessing of a highly bred racial stock" (P. 448, similar also P. 493). "A state which in this age of racial poisoning dedicates itself to the care of its best racial elements must some day become lord of the earth." (P. 782)

Hitler seems to have in mind a special stimulation of the nordic racial elements. The term "nordic race" does not, as far as I can see, appear in his book, but in several places he praises the "aryans" and places the Jews as their opposite. The Jews are made responsible — certainly too one-sided and in an exaggerated manner — for almost all of today's manifestations of decomposition. The Jews, so Hitler, says, lack "the most essential requirement for a cultured people, the idealistic attitude", they possess "no kind of culture-forming strength." (P. 332) The excellence of the "aryan" in comparison to this dark background shines in an even brighter light. "Everything we admire on this earth today — science and art, technology and inventions — are the creative product of only a few races, and originally perhaps of one race. On them depends the existence of this whole culture. If they perish, the beauty of this earth will sink into the grave with them." "All great cultures of the past perished only because the original creative race died out from blood poisoning." (P. 316) "The racial question gives the key not only to world history, but to all human culture." (P. 372) Hitler was obviously influenced by H. S. Chamberlain, indirectly possibly by Gobineau, who also did not like the Jews, but who was more just to them. But he seems to have taken some ideas from Th. Fritsch. An influence of Gunther's on Hitler's book is less obvious, but it may be presumed that he read Günther also. Just as did Gobineau and Chamberlain, Hitler exaggerates the harmful consequences of racial mixing. "Blood mixture and the resultant drop in the racial level is the sole cause of the death of old cultures; for men do not perish as a result of lost wars but by the loss of that force of resistance which is contained only in good blood." (P. 324, similarly also on P. 442 and 443) In other places, of course, he also shows understanding of the restriction of selection as a cause for degeneration (e.g. P. 145) and for the real decisive cause of decay, contre-selection e.g. on P. 582 and P. 583, where he talks about the selective effect of war. The principal significance of selection for the forming of races and species is stressed on P. 144/145 and p. 313.

In fact, it is rather important that racial hygiene must make a point of the preservation and advancement of those racial elements which created our culture. 'Thus the highest purpose of a racial state is concern for the preservation of those original elements which bestow culture and create the beauty and dignity of a higher mankind." (P. 434) But it depends how "the attempt to support above all those elements recognised as especially racially valuable basic elements inside the racial community, and to especially care for their increase" (P. 493) is carried out practically. Hitler thought of border colonies, "whose inhabitants are exclusively bearers of the highest racial purity and hence of the highest racial efficiency." (P. 449) "Specially constituted racial commissions must issue settlement certificates to individuals. For this, however, definite racial purity must be established." (P. 448) But in a mixed population such as ours it is not possible to establish, based on external characteristics, the affiliation of the major part of the hereditary mass. Blond hair does not vouch for aristocratic race, dark hair does not exclude it. In relation to social selection Hitler remarks very appropriately: "This sifting as to ability and efficiency cannot be done mechanically, but it is work which the fight for daily life takes care of all the time." (P. 493) This trial in daily life is, in my opinion, the best measure for racial hygienic selection. Naturally the party book may not be used as a measure for efficiency. An example of racial downfall to Hitler is France, which he does not like in any respect. This, according to Hitler, "makes such rapid progress in its negrification, that one can actually speak of the formation of an African state on European ground." (P. 730) This may be a little exaggerated, but the danger threatening France directly and the whole of Europe indirectly is seen correctly all the same. When he speaks of the "Frenchdom which is dying out not only in its population but especially in its best racial elements" (P. 766) he seems not to have been aware of the fact, that the present number of children of the German race is even less sufficient for preservation than that of the French.

Hitler strongly supports sterilisation of the inferior. "The demand that it should be made impossible for defective people to beget any offspring is a demand which is clearly reasonable and in its planned execution is the most humane deed (action) of mankind. It will save millions of the unfortunate poeple their undeserved sufferings, and as a result will lead to a raising of health on the whole." (P. 279) From the fact that he speaks of millions of unfortunates, it is evident that he demands sterilisation not only in extreme cases, which would be rather ineffective for the improvement of the health of the race, but that he wishes it to include the whole of the inferior part of the population.

He appreciates the significance of an early marriage to its full extent. "To be sure, it can be made possible only by quite a number of social conditions without which early marriage is not even thinkable." (P. 276) He quite appreciates the fact that a solution to this question is not possible without decisive social measures. One can expect that the national socialist movement will actively stand up for a compensation of family expenses.

The remarks about the increase of the demands on life, which is a major reason for the excessive restriction of births, are very much to the point. "The demands of people concerning food and clothing are increasing from year to year and now bear no relation to say, the demands of our forefathers one hundred years ago." (P. 146) As the increase of the demands is to a great extent caused by the extravagance of those who are childless, an effective compensation of family expenses would be achieved by down scaling the exaggerated increase of demands. "Certainly at a certain time all of mankind will be forced to discontinue the propagation of the human species due to the impossibility of aligning the fertility of the soil with the still rising population number." (P. 147) A race, however, which advances with the attitude of propagation will eliminate itself.

One important prerequisite for the preservation of the racial basis of our nation is an education designed in this manner. "The whole of the work in education and cultivation in a racial state must see its climax in burning in racial purpose and racial feeling instinctively and rationally into the hearts and brains of our youth" (P. 475). "The purpose of female education is to become a future mother." (P. 460) The young brain should not generally be strained with things it 90 % does not need. (P. 460) The teaching of French in the upper schools should be removed. (P. 465) The material in history classes should be substantially shortened (P. 467) ; in history the dominant position should be held by racial questions. (P. 468) If the superfluous and therefore very damaging jumble of education would be removed from the schools, then, I would like to add, it would be possible to shorten the whole period of the upper schools by two years which would be urgently desirable in view of the intent to encourage early marriages.

Just as important a task of the education system, as is the upbringing, is the social selection or as Hitler calls it "human selection." (P. 477) The racial state does "not have the task of maintaining the controlling influence of the existing class of society, but the task of extracting from the sum of all racial comrades the most capable heads and to bring them to office and position." (P. 480) But the racial hygienist must ensure that these able heads do not by their very rising die out as they have done." Hitler cannot stand the thought "that every year hundreds of thousands of totally inactive people are honoured with a higher education, whereas hundreds of thousands of others who have high aptitude receive no higher education." (P. 479) However, Hitler seems to have too optimistic an opinion as regards the frequency of high mental aptitude among the lower classes. Here I refer to the conclusions of Hartnackes (Natural Laws on Mental Education, Leipzig 1930).

Hitler is not afraid to point out unpopular truths. He comments about the alcohol question : "If, for instance, a whole continent has finally declared war on alcohol poisoning, in order to get a race out of the claws of this destructive vice, then suddenly our European bourgeois world has nothing left but an insignificant stare and a headshake and a superior feeling of ridicule — which looks especially well in this ridiculous society." (P. 450) In other cases he also names the things by their correct name: "Our whole public life today is like a hothouse of sexual ideas and temptations. One need only look at the menu of our cinemas, varieties and theatres, and one can hardly deny that this is not the right diet, especially for the young." (P. 278)

External politics also has a purpose, "to ensure the existence of the race which is embraced by the state." (P. 728) If Germany in 1904 had done what Japan did, then a world war would have been prevented. "Had blood been shed in 1904 it would have saved ten times as much blood in the years 1914-1918." (P. 155) For this the friendship of England would have been required. Therefore, Germany should have relinquished colonies and sea-power to concentrate all power of the state into a land-force (P. 154, similar also P. 753). The so-called "risk-idea" by Tirpitz was stated to be totally incorrect (P. 300). "I admit openly that even prior to the war I thought it would be more correct, if Germany had relinquished its stupid colonial policy, and having relinquished its trade and war fleet, then united with England against Russia, and in so doing would have gone from a weak commonplace policy to a strong determined European policy of continental land acquisition." (P. 753) I can only agree with these conclusions and have so stated several times (e.g. B.F.L. Bd II P. 396/397).

Hitler believes that such a policy will again be possible in the future, and in this sense he wants to give the German race a "political testament," a large goal, upon which external politics is to be oriented without being damaged by possible decisions of the day. "We stop the eternal Germanic trek to the South and West of Europe, and direct the view towards the land in the East. We finally stop the pre-war colonial and trade policy and move over towards the land policy of the future." (P. 742) The development of world economics in the years since Hitler wrote his book shows our people the same direction. We will simply be forced to seek our basis for life mainly in the country. "Even the possibility of a healthy farming class as a foundation for the whole nation can never be estimated highly enough. Many of our sufferings today are only the consequences of an unhealthy relationship between the country and the town populace." (P. 157)

Such a policy would also cause a community interest of all large Germanic races all by itself, which is not only desirable for ideological reasons but which follows from a well understood interest in life of the Germanic races. "One should not permit oneself to be torn by the differences of the individual people of a larger racial community. The fight which rages today is about very large goals: a culture fighting for its existence which combines millenia and embraces Greekdom and Germanism equally." (P. 470)

Hitler directs himself sharply against the demands of the restoration of the German borders of 1914, which he calls a political nonsense of dimensions and results, which make it seem a crime. Apart from the fact that for such a policy the means of power are absent, they would, even if undertaken successfully, lead to a further bleeding to death of our racial body, for which no responsibility could be taken. Especially South Tyrol must be deliberately sacrificed as we cannot do without either the friendship of Italy or England. With respect to possible future wars, Hitler says: "Diplomacy must ensure that a race does not perish heroically, but is maintained practically." (P. 693) "Even today we still dream of a heroism which robbed our people of millions of its most royal blood bearers, but the end result was totally barren." (P. 735) Today the means of power of the German Reich are so poor, that a fight against France would only be a slaughter of German youth; and the end result would be the unalterable defeat and the end of the German Reich.

In a future war the technical equipment will be more decisive than the number of soldiers. (P. 748) By this sentence one of his earlier sentences is corrected in which he says about the winning back of external power : "The prerequisites of this are not, however, arms as our bourgeois 'statesmen' prattle about, but the power of will." (P. 365) In this respect the 'bourgeois' statesmen seemed not to be too wrong. And they were especially right compared to the Hitler of 1923, who had forgotten that. Had Hitler had greater success at the beginning, then France would not have missed the opportunity to shoot down the rest of the German youth, and would have achieved its goal, which Hitler also acknowledges, the destruction of the German Reich. One can surely understand that Hitler's national enthusiasm had led him to take that step at that time, which he would hardly have done if he had let "reason as the only leader" bear on him, which he expresses as a fundamental rule on Page 753. Probably today he knows himself, that it was better for the existence of the Reich that his insurgence was suppressed right in its beginnings. A person with cancer must definitely risk an operation even where there is only one half a percent chance of a successful outcome (P. 463); but even Hitler will have to admit that chances for success today are better than they were and that there is justifiable hope that they will get better still. And he himself has today and in the future a better chance of significantly partaking in this salvation than he had then.

Hitler's ability in influencing the masses is admirable. He talks of the ways and means of mass influence with startling frankness. "Propaganda is to be used on the broad public in content and form, and its correctness is to be measured exclusively in its effective result." (P. 376) "As long as the realization of the mass remains as small as it is now and the state remains as indifferent as it is today, the masses will always follow that person first, who offers the most impertinent promises in economic matters." (P. 354) Poison will only be overcome by anti-poison. One may presume that Hitler knows exactly that a race cannot live on anti-poison. "I do not measure the speech of a statesman by the impression it left in a professor of a university, but by the effect it creates on the people." (P. 534) One will constantly have to be aware of this factor, when one reads certain remarks of Hitler about economic demands, about possibilities of external politics and also about the Jewish question over which one sometines just shakes onés head...

s ist ein tragisches Geschick, daß Ploetz die Lösung des Problems der
'erständigung und Zusammenarbeit der nordischen Völker nicht mehr er-
ebte, er, der an die zielbewußte Führung Adolf Hitlers, an dessen heili-
e, nationale und internationale rassenhygienische Mission so felsenfest
laubte. Aber es mag ein Trost für uns sein, daß er bis zu seinem letzten
.temzuge in unerschütterlicher Hoffnung am Waffensieg des deutschen Vol-
es und im darauffolgendem Frieden am Glauben an den weiteren Sieges-
ug auch der Rassenhygiene festhielt.

Rüdin.

It is tragic that Ploetz did not live to see the solution of the problem of understanding and cooperation amongst the Nordic races, when he believed so ardently in the purposeful leadership of Adolf Hitler, and in his holy, national and international racial hygienic mission. But let it be a consolation to us that until his last breath he maintained the unshakeable hope of a victory of conquest of the German race and that in the then ensuing peace there would follow a victory in racial hygiene.

E. Rüdin

Rüdin acknowledges Hitler's zeal in learning about racial hygiene in Ploetz's obituary.

WORLD FEDERATION FOR MENTAL HEALTH
MEMBER ASSOCIATIONS AND AFFILIATED ORGANISATIONS 1970

MEMBER ASSOCIATIONS

ARGENTINA
Liga Argentina de Higiene Mental
Fundacion Argentina para la Salud Mental (F.A.S.A.M.)

ARUBA
Aruba Society for Mental Health

AUSTRALIA
The Australian and New Zealand College of Psychiatrists
New South Wales Association for Mental Health
Victorian Council for Mental Hygiene
Western Australian Mental Health Association (Inc.)

AUSTRIA
Oesterreichische Gesellschaft für Psychische Hygiene

BELGIUM
Ligue Nationale Belge d'Hygiène Mentale
Association Catholique d'Hygiène Mentale
Fédération des Institutions Hospitalières de Caritas Catholica
Fondation Julie Renson
Fondation Nationale Reine Fabiola pour la Santé Mentale

CANADA
Canadian Mental Health Association
Canadian Psychiatric Association
Canadian Psychological Association

CEYLON
Ceylon Mental Health Association

CHILE
Asociacion Chiltena Pro Salud Mental

CHINA (Taiwan)

COSTA RICA
Chinese Nacional Association for Mental Health
Comite Nacional de Salud Mental

CUBA
Sociedad Cubana de Psiquiatria

CYPRUS
Pancyprian Society for Mental Health

CZECHOSLOVAKIA
Psychiatric Section of the Czechoslovak Medical Society
J. E. Purkynre Sokolska 3i, Praha, 2

DENMARK
Landsforeningen for Mentalhygiejne

FINLAND
Suomen Mielenterveysseura

FRANCE
Ligue Française d'Hygiène Mentale
Association "l'Elan Retrouvé"
Association Française pour la Sauvegarde de l'Enfance et l'Adolescence
Centre Technique National pour l'Enfance et l'Adolescence Inadaptees
Comite National Français de Défense contre l'Alcoolisme
Ecole des Parents et des Educateurs
Federation Française des Travailleurs Sociaux
Federation des Societes de Medicine Psychosomatique
Societe Française de Medecine Psychosomatique

GERMAN DEMOCRATIC REPUBLIC
Gesellschaft für Ärztliche Psychotherapie der DDR

GERMAN FEDERAL REPUBLIC
Arbeitsgemeinschaft für Seelische Gesundheit (Psychohygiene)

UNITED STATES OF AMERICA and its Territories
The National Association for Mental Health, Inc.
The American Society of Psychoanalytic Medicine
Academy of Religion and Mental Health
The American Academy of Psychoanalysis
American Association on Mental Deficiency
American Child Guidance Foundation, Inc.
The American Foundation for Mental Hygiene, Inc.
The American Foundation of Religion and Psychiatry
American Group Psychotherapy Association, Inc.
American Medical Association
American Neurological Association
American Occupational Therapy Association
The American Orthopsychiatric Association, Inc.
American Psychiatric Association
American Psychoanalytic Association
American Psychological Association
American Psychosomatic Society
American Society of Adlerian Psychology
American Society for Clinical Hypnosis
Association for the Advancement of Psychoanalysis, Inc.
Association for the Advancement of Psychotherapy
Association for Group Psychoanalysis and Process, Inc.
Austen Riggs Center, Inc.
Chestnut Lodge, Inc.
Child Study Association of America
Elwyn Institute
Grainick Foundation
Group for the Advancement of Psychiatry, Inc.
The Hogg Foundation for Mental Health
The Institute for Research in Hypnosis
The Morton Prince Clinic for Hypnotherapy
Jewish Board of Guardians
The Menninger Foundation
Mental Health Film Board, Inc.
National Association for Retarded Children
National Association of Social Workers, Inc.
National Psychological Association for Psychoanalysis, Inc.
Postgraduate Center for Mental Health, Inc.
William Alanson White Psychoanalytic Society

VIRGIN ISLANDS
St. Thomas Mental Health Association

URUGUAY
Liga Nacional contra el Alcoholismo

VENEZUELA
Liga Venezolana de Higiene Mental

YUGOSLAVIA
National Association for the Mentally Handicapped in SFR Yugoslavia

TRANS-NATIONAL ASSOCIATIONS
(listed in order of admission to membership)

International Association for Child Psychiatry and Allied Professions
Ligue Européenne d'Hygiène Mentale
Association Latino-Americana Pro Salud Mental
International Psycho-Analytical Association
Bureau International Catholique de l'Enfance (BICE)
International Council of Psychologists
International Society for General Semantics
International Association of Individual Psychology

MALTA
The Malta Welfare Society for the Mentally Handicapped

NETHERLANDS
Federatie van Instellingen voor de Zorg voor Alcoholisten
Universitaire Boekhandel Nederland Medische Boekhandel
Foundation for Alcoholstudies
Hervormde Stichting voor Geestelijke, Volksgezondheid voor Amsterdam en Omgeving
Katholiek Nationaal Bureau voor Geestelijke Gezondheidzorg
Medische Consultatie bureau voor alcoholisme
Nationaal Protestants Centrum voor de Geestelijke Volksgezondheid
N.V. Philips-Gloeilampenfabrieken Gezondheidscentrum
Stichting Algemeen Centraal Bureau voor de Geestelijke Volksgezondheid

NEW ZEALAND
The Canterbury Association for Mental Health
Otago Association for Mental Health

SENEGAL
Societe de Psychopathologie et d'Hygiene Mentale de Dakar

SOUTH AFRICA, Republic of
Cape Mental Health Society
Mental Health Society of the Witwatersrand
Port Elizabeth Mental Health Society

SWITZERLAND
Clinique Bellevue
Clinique Psychiatrique "La Metairie"
Clinique "Viannetto"
Federation internationale des Services de Secours Par Telephone
J. R. Geigy S.A.
Les Laboratoires Sapos S.A.
Gemeinschaft für Psychologie Zusammenschluss von Psychologisch Ausgebildeten (Akademikern)
Vereinigung der Schweizerischen Psychologen (VSP)

UNITED ARAB REPUBLIC
Behman Hospital

UNITED KINGDOM
Birmingham (Mental A)
Hospital Management Committee
Board of Management for Crichton Royal Hospital
Darenth Park Hospital
Hampstead Child Therapy Course and Clinic
Hardmanfast Hospital
Manchester Regional Hospital Board
May and Baker Ltd
Moorhaven Hospital Management Committee
North Wales Hospital
Board of Management for Paisley and District Hospitals
Smith Kline & French Laboratories Ltd
Stallington Hospital Management Committee
St. Bernard's Hospital Management Committee
St. Lawrence's Hospital Management Committee
The Administrative Staff College
The Bethlem Royal Hospital and the Maudsley Hospital
The Mental After Care Association
The National Hospitals for Nervous Diseases
The Uffculme Clinic
Warlingham Park Hospital Management Committee

UNITED STATES OF AMERICA
Alfred Adler Mental Hygiene Clinic
American Mental Health Foundation, Inc.
American Institute for Research in the Behavioral Sciences
American Institute of Family Relations

148

GREECE
The Athenian Institute of Anthropos
Center for Mental Health and Research
Hellenic Society of Neurology and Psychiatry
Panhellenic Union for Mental Hygiene
GUATEMALA
Liga Guatemalteca de Higiene Mental
HONG KONG
Mental Health Association of Hong Kong
ICELAND
Icelandic Mental Health Association
INDIA
Indian Psychiatric Society
The Indian Council for Mental Hygiene
National Organisation for the Protection of Children (N.O.P.C.)
IRAN
Persian Federation for Mental Health
IRELAND
The Mental Health Association of Ireland
ISRAEL
Israel Association for Mental Health
ITALY
Lega Italiana d'Igiene e Profilassi Mentale
Società Italiana per l'Assistenza Medico-Psico-Pedagogica
JAPAN
Japan Association for Mental Health
Japan Federation for Mental Health
LEBANON
Lebanese Society of Neurology and Psychiatry
MAURITIUS
Mauritius Mental Health Association
MEXICO
Liga Mexicana de Salud Mental
NETHERLANDS
Nationale Federatie voor de Geestelijke Volksgezondheid
NORWAY
Norges Landsforening for Mentalhygiene
PAKISTAN
Pakistan Institute for Mental Hygiene
PERU
Liga Peruana de Higiene Mental
PHILIPPINES
Philippine Mental Health Association, Inc.
POLAND
Polskie Towarzystwo Higieny Psychicznej
PORTUGAL
Associacao de Pais e Amigos das Crianças Diminuidas Mentais
Liga Portuguesa de Higiene Mental
SOUTH AFRICA, Republic of
The South African National Council for Mental Health
SPAIN
Instituto de Medicina Psicologica
SUDAN, Republic of the
The Sudan National Association for Mental Health
SWEDEN
Svensa Foreningen for Psykisk Halsovard
SWITZERLAND
Association Suisse pour la Protection de la Sante Mentale
Pro Infirmis
THAILAND
Mental Health Association of Thailand
TURKEY
Turkish Association for Mental Hygiene
UNITED ARAB REPUBLIC
Egyptian Association for Mental Health
UNITED KINGDOM
Association of Child Psychotherapists (Non-Medical)
British Psychological Society
Federation of Associations of Mental Health Workers
The Institute of Dental Psychology Ltd.
Mental Health Research Fund
National Association of Chief Male Nurses
National Society for Mentally Handicapped Children
The Northern Ireland Association for Mental Health
The Richmond Fellowship

AFFILIATED ORGANIZATIONS

AUSTRALIA
Reparation Department Psychiatric Service
BELGIUM
Assistance Publique de Liège
Centre d'Études des Relations Humaines et de leur Perfectionnement
CIDAR, Centre pour la Recherche Anthropologique Interdisciplinaire
Clinique Psychiatrique Universitaire
CANADA
Brown Camps Residential & Day Schools Operating as Browndale
Canadian Psychoanalytic Society
Centre d'Information sur l'Enfance et l'Adolescence Inadaptées
Order Division Library, University of Guelph
Hospital Saint-Charles de Joliette
Ontario Association for the Mentally Retarded
Ontario Teacher's Federation
Université de Sherbrooke
CEYLON
The Rotherfield Psychological Society
CZECHOSLOVAKIA
League for the Ministry of Heart
FRANCE
"Arc-en-Ciel"
Association d'Entraide "Vivre"
Association d'Etudes et de Recherches et l'Education Surveillée
Centre Henri Rousselle
Centre de Posture et de Réadaptation Scolaire Agricole de l'Ouest
Centre de Psychiatrie Sociale
Centre Psychothérapique Barthélemy-Durand
Federation Nationale des Departements de Montfavet
L'Union Nationale des Amis et Parents de Malades Mentaux
Hôpital Psychiatrique "Bon Sauveur"
Hôpital Psychiatrique de Château Picon
Hôpital Psychiatrique "La Grimaudière"
Hôpital Psychiatrique de Vaucluse
Institut Coopératif de l'École Moderne
Maison de Santé St. Vincent de Paul
Société Française de Psychologie
UNAPEI - Union Nationale des Associations de Parents d'Enfance Inadaptés
GERMANY
Arbeitskreis Neue Erziehung E.V.
Institut fuer Psychohygiene e.V.
Institut fuer Erziehungshilfe E.V.
Studiengemeinschaft fuer praktische Psychologie E.V.
GREECE
Dromosi Foundation Mental Hospital
Ormona Foundation for the Rehabilitation of the Disabled
HONG KONG
New Life Psychiatric Rehabilitation Association
INDIA
The Society for the Care, Treatment and Training of Children in Need
of Special Care
IRELAND
St. Patrick's Hospital
ISRAEL
AKIM, Israeli Association for Rehabilitation of the Mentally
Handicapped
Jewish National & Library
ITALY
A.M.I.S.I., Associazione Medica Italiana per lo Studio dello Ipnosi
Associazione "Eugenio Medea" Pro Infanzia Anormale Sezione
Lombarda Della S.I.A.M.E.
Centro d'Igiene Mentale
Centro d'Igiene Mentale
Centro di Incontri e di Collaborazione
Clinica delle Malattie Nervose e Mentali dell'Università di Genova
Instituto di Indagini Psicologiche
Istituto Neuropsichiatrico Provinciale di Firenze
JAPAN

Foundlin House Foundation, Inc.
Geneva State Hospital School
The Netherlands Organisation "GROW"
Grove School
Harbor General Hospital
Hillside Hospital
Indiana Assoc. for Health & Welfare, Inc.
Individual Psychology Assoc. New York Inc.
Institute for Intercultural Studies
Institute for Rational Living, Inc.
Junior Chamber International
Lafayette Clinic
Lincoln Institute for Psychotherapy
Long Island Consultation Center
Maryland Assoc. for Private Psychiatrists
McLean Hospital
Mental Health Assoc. of the Cincinnati Area, Inc.
Mental Health Assoc. of Westchester County, Inc.
Mental Health Society of Greater Chicago, Inc.
Methodist Hospital of Gary, Inc.
Milwaukee County Mental Health Assoc.
Mental Health Assoc. of Central Connecticut
National Assoc. for Music Therapy, Inc.
National Association of Private Psychiatric Hospitals
National Assoc. of Psychiatric Technology
New York Psychoanalytic Institute
NIMH Of Library
NISH Of Library
Philadelphia Child Guidance Clinic
Philadelphia Mental Health Clinic
Psychiatric Clinic, Student Health Service, U.C.L.A. Medical Centre
Psychiatric Research Foundation of Cleveland
Read-More Publications
School Guidance Center, Inc.
Social Dept. & Mental Hygiene Clinic
San Fernando Valley State College
Suicide Prevention Center
The Guidance Center (of Springfield Ohio)
State Univ. of New York at Stony Brook
The Powell School at Home for Mentally Handicapped
The Psychoneurose Research Foundation
The Seton Psychiatric Institute
University Hospital, Psychiatric Inst.
Univ. of South Florida
Washington Psychiatric Society
Western Illinois University
The Neuropsychiatric Institute
Albert Einstein Medical Center

INTERNATIONAL
Christian Psychiatric Center, Inc.
International Centre for Genetic Education
International Community Mental Health Seminars
International Council for Children's Play
International Council of Jewish...
Pflege- u. Sozialarbeitern in der Nervenheilkunde, e.V.
International Society for Clinical and Experimental Hypnosis
Società Internazionale de Psychologia dell'Espressione
Centro Internazionale di Ignosi Medica e Psicologica

www.ingramcontent.com/pod-product-compliance
Lightning Source LLC
Chambersburg PA
CBHW070825100426
42813CB00003B/492